THE WHISTLE-BLOWER

THE WHISTLE-BLOWER

Joanna Seldon

The University of Buckingham Press

Published in 2017 by

The University of Buckingham Press
Yeomanry House
Hunter Street
Buckingham MK18 1EG

A CIP catalogue record for this book is available at the British Library

ISBN 978-1-908684-974

Printed in the United Kingdom by Henry Ling Limited, at the Dorset Press, Dorchester, DT1 1HD

****

'May I never see in the patient anything but a fellow creature in pain'

(Moses Maimonides, twelfth century CE rabbi and physician; the epigraph to
Maurice Pappworth's 'Human Guinea Pigs')

'Do unto others as you would have them do unto you.'

(the 'Golden Rule': Leviticus, 19:18; Matthew, 7:12)

*'I will use my power to help the sick to the best of my ability and judge-
ment; I will abstain from harming or wronging any man by it.'*

(from the Hippocratic Oath, fifth to third centuries BCE, translated from the
Greek by J. Chadwick and W.N. Mann)

*'The voluntary consent of the human subject is absolutely essential.
This means that the person involved should have legal capacity to give
consent; should be so situated as to be able to exercise free power of
choice, without the intervention of any element of force, fraud, deceit,
duress, over-reaching, or other ulterior form of constraint or coercion;
and should have sufficient knowledge and comprehension of the elements of the subject matter involved as to enable him to make an understanding and enlightened decision...*

*The experiment should be such as to yield fruitful results for the good
of society, unprocurable by other methods or means of study, and not
random and unnecessary in nature...*

*The experiment should be so conducted as to avoid all unnecessary
physical and mental suffering and injury...'*

(from the 1947 Nuremberg Code, a set of ethical principles for human experimentation created after the post-war trial of Nazi physicians)

Contents

Foreword

Unearthing wrong doing, criticising the actions of others and demanding change are difficult enough tasks at the best of times. However when the object of the challenge is the leadership of a professional body, one is part of that profession, the profession is medicine and the time is the post war decades, 'difficult' does not begin to describe the task faced by the protagonist.

Such men and women have great intellect and foresight and of course by definition, personal courage in abundance. They are also, often outsiders and members of the 'awkward squad' but that squad tends to have only one member. Maurice Pappworth is a frighteningly well worked example of this caricature, the brilliant outsider who sacrificed career for a truth that many saw but only he was prepared to put his head above the parapet and get it shot off, and that is exactly what the medical establishment did to him.

At the core of this story is the clash between a little Jew brought up in poor circumnstances, who came from Liverpool rather than London, had none of the requisite charms or behaviours apparently required, was revered by his students but dismissed by a powerful establishment of academics who knew everything but understood nothing. The author Joanna Seldon was Pappworth's daughter and was herself a remarkable woman who was able to both talk and write about her father with great candour. She loved and admired him but could also see his weaknesses and frailties which she records without justification or excuse.

This text is more warning than narrative. There are still controversies over the ethics and conduct of some trials particularly but not exclusively, in relation to those performed in the developing world where standards of care are not the same as in the countries of the trial sponsors. We must remain forever questioning of ourselves and each other that whatever experiments or clinical trials we are engaged with, we do not compromise patient autonomy or exploit their vulnerability whether they live the Surrey Hills or rural Indian.

Pappworth's life story reminds us to that prejudice is never far away. The anti-Semitism Pappworth undoubtedly encountered as a medical student, during the war and in the 50s and 60s, did not disappear in the 1970s rather, it changed its focus and the targets became women, doctors from the gay community and those of Indian, Pakistani or Sri Lankan decent. Today I look at the leadership of my profession and in particular as the child of immigrants myself, the children of the latter group of doctors who are now so prominent in their fields and can't help thinking that maybe, just maybe some of Pappworth's fight is won.

Professor Martin Gore CBE PhD FRCP
Consultant Medical Oncologist and Professor of Cancer Medicine
The Royal Marsden NHS Foundation Trust and The Institute of Cancer Research, London.

Preface by Sir Anthony Seldon

Joanna devoted herself with extraordinary courage and focus to writing this book on her father in 2016, the last year of her life. She summoned the strength for a journey we made to Poland, to see the village where her father's family had lived. I cannot remember exactly when the seed of writing his biography formed in her mind, but she had always been immensely inspired by him, and believed he had not been fairly treated by colleagues in the medical profession. In particular, she was immensely proud of his book, *Human Guinea Pigs*, which was published in 1967, shortly before her 13th birthday. It was as if, in her biography, she sought for him an acceptance and respect for his work which he never fully achieved in his lifetime. When she became ill five years ago with her inoperable cancer, she began to reflect upon his powers as a medic, and wondered what advice and solace he might have given to her. One of her last poems was written to him, and runs thus:

My Father
Who healed the sick,
Now too far away
To heal me,
Stir your spirit
To remind me
What it is to live
The best that can be
Lived
So long as I am
Here.

Preface by Joanna Seldon

It was the night of 20 February 2012. I was lying in my bed at the Royal Marsden Hospital in London feeling anxious and rather frightened about the procedure I was to undergo the following morning. The chemo-embolization of my liver was considered to be the best way of treating the neuro-endocrine tumour diagnosed eight months earlier, which had at some point metastasised to my liver. It had all been carefully explained to me. In order to cut off the blood supply to the tumour and, it was hoped, reduce it, a catheter would be passed through my groin and into the liver, carrying several beads of chemotherapy. I would be given just a local anaesthetic, and remain conscious throughout. The subsequent pain, I was assured, wouldn't be too bad, although the chemotherapy would have some unpleasant side-effects.

On the subject of catheters I was a little hazy. The first (and possibly only) time I had encountered the word before was when, aged thirteen in 1967, I succeeded in reading, cover to cover, *Human Guinea Pigs:* my father Dr Maurice Pappworth's controversial, whistle-blowing book about unethical experimentation on humans. For me, the summer of 1967 was significant. I was awarded my Junior Work Badge and was batmitzvah (the girls' equivalent to barmitzvah – only recently introduced at our synagogue). For my father, May 1967 marked the culmination of fifteen years' work as he tracked and noted the dubious direction of British medicine – notably, in the hallowing of clinical research over patient care.

The message I remembered from *Human Guinea Pigs* was that catheters are invasive, and you never quite know where they're going to end up. Pulling myself higher onto my pillows, making sure I wasn't disturbing the drip machine, I told myself to calm down and listen to something soothing on my iPod. No-one had yet disturbed me to do my observations or measure out my nighttime meds; everything at that point seemed peaceful and still.

It was then that my father visited me. I don't believe in ghosts, and I'm not at all sure what I think about the after-life. But there can be absolutely no doubt that, at that moment, I felt the presence of my father more strongly than I ever had since his death nearly eighteen years earlier in 1994. Maurice Pappworth, the physician-friend, was watching over me. I saw nothing; I heard nothing; I was simply overwhelmed, just for a minute or two, by the sense that he was there in that hospital room with me – as he had been with countless anxious patients for more than half a century. Was he there to tell me everything would be all right? Call that wishful thinking, if you like. Suffice to say that, after the procedure, I enjoyed two years of good health (although I had been completely misled about pain levels, which I remember finding comparable to childbirth).

I haven't had a similar encounter with my late father since that February night, even though I have been in hospital on a number of occasions since. But what that experience taught me (and I think it was a deeply spiritual one) is that central to the care of the sick is the gentle presence of the physician. Theirs is a relationship based not on power and vulnerability but on empathy and trust. This idea was central to Maurice Pappworth's thinking, and it spurred him to write the book which compromised his career. It is a fascinating story, and so I decided to write it.

Introduction

When doctors become torturers: why the whistle had to blow

'When the saturation of oxygen fell to below 40 per cent, the infants began to move and become restless, finally crying strenuously, sometimes in a gasping fashion. One infant had a period of apnoea (cessation of breathing).'

(Report on an experiment in oxygen deprivation carried out in Boston in 1961 on infants under one year old; cited in Maurice Pappworth's 'Human Guinea Pigs')

'I don't like what I'm being asked to do.'

It had obviously taken some courage for the junior doctor studying for his Membership exam for the Royal College of Physicians (MRCP) to approach his tutor, though Dr Maurice Pappworth was the least forbidding of pedagogues: just a few inches over five feet tall, with twinkly blue eyes and a slightly eccentric sense of humour. But it is never easy telling tales, especially if your professional seniors are implicated. Especially, perhaps, if those professionals are doctors. Maurice Pappworth was to experience this truth at considerable personal cost.

'What are you being asked to do?' Pappworth had encountered other such nervous approaches from his MRCP students in the 1950s and 1960s, and he had a fairly clear idea that the young man's anxiety would be on the same subject. Whenever Pappworth mentioned to his postgraduate students – and they will have caught the irony in his tone – 'recent medical advances', one or two would sidle up to him at the end of the class. They wanted to tell their teacher about unethical experiments they had personally observed in the British hospitals where they worked or were attending courses. For them, the dilemma was a difficult one: should they play a role in persuading a patient to volunteer, knowing that failure to co-operate might jeopardise their career?

The evidence Pappworth had started to gather all pointed to a gradual lapse in the medical profession, away from the ethical values outlined in the ancient Hippocratic Oath and the very recent Nuremberg Code of 1947. In essence,

1

these protected the needs and dignity of the patient. The needs and ambitions of doctors, and of the organisations that represent them, were secondary. Maurice Pappworth, a great teacher and clinician, never ceased to put the patient first. It distressed him to hear and read of colleagues who failed to share that priority. The whole issue of how doctors should regard those in their care became focused on the *cause celebre* of Pappworth's career: the 'human guinea pigs' caged in our hospitals, subjects of medical research and, in the way they were treated as such, the touchstone of our moral values. Pappworth, already an outsider, was prepared to push himself further into the cold. He was going to tell the world what was going on.

Now was the time to do it, for the demystification of medicine began in the 1960's. By this decade medicine had started to change, developing well beyond a simple diagnosis and a few treatments. Hence, argued researchers, the need for randomised trials. But alongside this 'progress' came increasingly invasive procedures, and surgeons were keen to keep pushing for the heights without restriction.

Stricter oversight was therefore clearly required at this point: zealous enthusiasm, and the prospect of ever more daring techniques, should not be allowed to triumph over honesty, compassion and professional decency. Drug companies were naturally in favour of thorough trials, to reduce the chance of their being sued. 1967, the year of publication of Pappworth's whistle-blowing book *Human Guinea Pigs*, was, according to medical historian and journalist Dr James Le Fanu, the high point of clinical research. As Pappworth prepared to write his book, he had the sense that it marked a change in part of the medical world, just as the atmosphere had changed during the twenty years since the Nuremberg Code.

As another medical historian, Jenny Hazelgrove, has pointed out, 'debates about research practices referred less to the Code than to traditional paternalistic ideals'. Although the Nuremberg judges who tried Nazi physicians placed great emphasis on the importance of informed consent, plenty of doctors remained determined to protect their research and ensure a steady supply of human subjects. It was those of his fellow 'paternalistic' professionals, who seemed to place the value of scientific discovery above the value of the human individual, that Pappworth decided to expose.

Pappworth was not alone in his concerns. Professor Andrew Ivy, an eminent American physiologist, physician and ethicist and the principal medical expert at the Nuremberg Trials, is credited with the wording of the Nuremberg

Code. While investigating experimentation on humans in 1966, Pappworth wrote to Ivy, whose reply stated that his own research work had always been rooted in the 'Golden Rule': do unto others as you would have them do to you. He wrote again a year later requesting a copy of Pappworth's newly-published *Human Guinea Pigs*: 'I am sure I shall profit by reading your book'. Indeed, Ivy himself is cited in it. Having emphasised that many of the doctors tried at Nuremberg for conducting horrific experiments were professors from the top of the German medical hierarchy, Pappworth quotes Ivy's contention: 'It is clear that several hundred more [Nazi doctors] were aware what was going on'.

Many British doctors during the 1950s and 1960s, though aware of the un-ethical research taking place in this country, nevertheless chose to turn a blind eye to it. Criticised, as we shall see, for the parallels he drew between the Third Reich and post-war Britain, Pappworth the 'enfant terrible' of medicine knew how to produce an effect. 'Not one of the convicted doctors', he reminds us, 'ever acknowledged that they had done anything wrong whatsoever or ex-pressed the slightest remorse.'

For them, the inmates of Auschwitz were, literally, a captive group on which to perform experiments 'far beyond normal limits'. He also quoted with approval the words of the German physician and physiologist Viktor von Weizsäcker from the appendix of the alarmingly titled book, *Doctors of Infamy*: 'There is not much difference whether a human being is looked upon as "a case" or as a number tattooed on the arm... This is the alchemy of the modern age, the transmogrification of subject into object, of man into a thing, against which our destructive urge may wreak its fury without restraint.'

Another doctor who shared Pappworth's concerns was Otto Guttentag of the University of California Medical School, who had fled Germany in 1933. It was he who coined the phrase "physician-friend", which so appealed to Pap-pworth that he used it at the end of *Human Guinea Pigs* to summarise what he saw as the crucial role of the doctor. He is the patient's trusted friend, rather than a curious scientist most interested in patients as potential research oppor-tunities. A friend is someone we trust, and it is the concept of trust between doctor and patient that dominated Pappworth's medical thinking – and one which is, fifty years after the publication of *Human Guinea Pigs*, as pertinent as ever. It is also one more generally recognised in an age when the professional classes are no longer seen as minor gods.

In his book, Pappworth details some of the experiments performed on the most vulnerable categories of patient. These included newborn babies. In one, carried out in a Toronto hospital in 1957, 'no sedative was given prior to the experiment'. During a 1963 experiment in California, the infants' feet were immersed in iced water for one minute. Aortic pressure was recorded during immersion and for two to five minutes afterwards. The report in the journal *Pediatrics* states that 'the infants invariably cried when exposed to cold'. What did the researchers expect?

In Philadelphia, an experiment involving two children aged three was described in the researcher's report as 'not devoid of difficulties'. In other words, it was potentially dangerous. He admits that the children 'required some restraint' – hardly surprising, given that their legs had been 'immobilized by bandaging them to a board'.

A 1961 report recounts an experiment on thirteen 'mentally deficient' infants under a year old, performed at an obstetrics and paediatric hospital in Boston. The researcher explains that the babies were given tightly-fitted face masks and deliberately subjected to hypoxia – oxygen deprivation – by inhaling a gas mixture of 90 per cent nitrogen, which is 'irrespirable'. 'When the saturation of oxygen fell to below 40 per cent, the infants began to move and become restless, finally crying strenuously, sometimes in a gasping fashion. One infant had a period of apnoea (cessation of breathing).' Pappworth doesn't need to comment. The experimenter's report reveals all that needs to be said about how abruptly medicine turns to cruelty.

An experiment at Taplow Hospital in Buckinghamshire in 1953 involved the deliberate blistering of the abdomens of forty-one children, aged between eight and fourteen, by the application of cantharides, an irritant. Pappworth quotes the doctor's description of the technique in the journal *Clinical Science*: 'Blister skin was removed with scissors, the raw area swabbed with peroxide and covered with oiled silk. Healing occurred in five to six days, leaving a small pigmented area.' He wonders whether these children were left permanently scarred.

The report in the *Journal of Obstetrics and Gynaecology* of an experiment at Edinburgh Royal Infirmary in 1949 on seventy-five pregnant women was pounced on by Pappworth. Cardiac catheterization was performed on them under X-ray control. 'The hazard of exposing pregnant women to radiation, especially in the early months, is not mentioned,' he observes. 'The report does mention, however, that three of the subjects were "obviously apprehensive".' Pappworth notes that some subjects were as young as fifteen.

One particularly gruesome experiment undertaken at Cincinnati General Hospital in 1951 involved giving pregnant women a high spinal anaesthetic. This induced temporary paralysis of the lower limbs, which will spread to the abdomen and chest if the patient is tilted. And tilted they were, the women remaining awake throughout. 'Spinal anaesthesia,' Pappworth remarks, 'is not a pleasant procedure for any patient and has well-recognised dangers. These become more likely the higher the paralysis is made to spread by the tilting.' In three of the five subjects, according to the researcher's report, the spinal anaesthetic reached the fourth cervical segment of the spinal cord. This, according to Pappworth, 'is very high and is likely to result in paralysis of the diaphragm.'

Twelve years later, at the Edinburgh Royal Infirmary, a group of women about to undergo Caesarean section were the subjects of a test to measure blood pressure in the inferior vena cava (a large vein that carries blood to the heart) in late pregnancy. A catheter and wire guide were passed along the femoral vein; then the catheter was moved up the vein as far as the right atrium of the heart. The women's pressures were recorded while they were placed in different positions from 'supine to lateral. The patients were then given a general anaesthetic and the pressure recordings were continued during the Caesarean operation.' The catheters were kept in position during the section, and before the abdomen was sutured (sewn up), 'the uterus was lifted forward by long stay sutures.'

The precise degree of risk, to either mother or baby, may not be easy to determine. 'But,' says Pappworth, 'the reader will judge whether, apart from risk of actual harm, pregnant women should be used in any of the ways described. In most societies a pregnant woman is given special consideration because of her condition. Surely such regard should be more common, not less, in medical circles.' One might argue that these experiments on pregnant women are an indication of the casual attitude and disregard for individual dignity shown in general to the female sex in the years prior to the revolution in attitudes of the 1960s and 1970s.

Pappworth's book is also exercised by experiments on patients suffering from heart conditions. For instance, some experimenters would deliberately induce heart stoppage in order to obtain better X-ray images. Cardiac arrest might be brought about by 'the injection of a powerful drug, acetylcholine, via the catheter, directly into the heart'. When this technique was performed on twenty-three patients at the Hahneman Hospital in Philadelphia in 1959, the period of cardiac arrest lasted from two to thirty-two seconds. Nine years earlier, an account in *Clinical Science* covered experiments at the Hammersmith Hospital in London performed on patients in their seventies (one, in fact, was over eighty) with heart failure. A large needle was kept in a main artery to take blood samples. 'It appears,' comments Pappworth, 'that doctors sometimes forget that those who are most in need of help, sympathy and gentle treatment are not the less sick but the most sick, and that among these the dying and the old have pre-eminent claims'. As always, he is championing the weak, and he cites instances of experiments performed on dying elderly people who passed away shortly afterwards, the experiment having speeded up the process.

Cancer patients are another vulnerable group whose subjection to unpleasant and generally non-therapeutic research is highlighted by Pappworth. At the University of California Medical School in 1955, patients with advanced cancer had hollow needles six inches long inserted directly into their livers; then catheters were passed through the needles to enter the hepatic or portal vein, where they stayed for between two and '*nineteen days*' (Pappworth's italics). The aim was to take numerous blood samples. Seventy-three patients described as 'seriously ill' took part. Pappworth comments that 'only in the case of two, who had cirrhosis of the liver, could the experiment be said to have direct relevance'. In three patients the needle accidentally pierced the bowel; in two it punctured a main artery, in another his gall bladder; one patient suffered from syncope (shock) and three had large haemorrhages.

Pappworth underlines time and again that experiments can go wrong. During a 1951 experiment, also carried out at the University of California Medical School and reported in the *American Journal of Roentgenology*, 'the physician became confused in the dark of the X-ray room and accidentally twisted the carotid artery into a knot'. As a result, the patient suffered a stroke twelve hours later.

He assembled evidence of these horrific abuses at a time, during the 1960s in particular, when the political establishment was being challenged by a new, counter-cultural generation, and the authority of the omniscient doctor was beginning to ebb. The interest shown by the media and the general public in Pappworth's exposure of dubious research practices – and, indeed, the steady closing of ranks against him by the medical establishment – were a symptom of the growing disaffection with the status quo. *Human Guinea Pigs*, published just over two-thirds into that most iconic of decades, arrived at a perfect moment.

Pappworth would spend many hours in the Royal Society of Medicine library, scanning journals in which seemingly unethical and possibly illegal experiments on humans were described. A key figure in helping Pappworth to compile his dossier of cases was Helen Bamber, whom he had first met at St George's Hospital, Wapping, in east London, where he was a temporary consultant, and she worked as an almoner and administrator. According to a profile of Bamber by Simon Hattenstone in *The Guardian*, she 'would help him with his administration, and they would talk in his rooms for hours about the overuse of drugs, unnecessary surgery, the Nazi doctors' malign experimentation.' Bamber, who at the age of twenty volunteered to go out and help after the relief of Bergen-Belsen concentration camp, went on to create the Medical Foundation for the Care of Victims of Torture (now the Helen Bamber Foundation). She remembered that Pappworth taught her about medical ethics as they worked together on *Human Guinea Pigs*. '"He was as preoccupied as I was with this question of total power, total helplessness." Together, they compiled an archive of abuses.'

In an interview with the research-ethics specialist Professor Allan Gaw in September 2011, three years before her death, Bamber recalled her first impressions of Maurice Pappworth: 'very small, compact... he had the capacity when he was talking about medicine to be very calm, although passionate at the same time. But when he was working there was a kind of very serious intent in him to get it right.' She admitted that putting together the case material for *Human Guinea Pigs* was 'disturbing... We discussed everything. He was a great one for explaining everything... He always wanted you to understand why he had those views and on what he based them... I understood him.' And she realised that he felt very 'pained' by the truths he was uncovering as he scoured the medical journals for evidence.

She sensed in him 'a mixture of courage to say what he felt was right, but a fear that it could really harm him'. A Jew herself, she touched in the interview on the question of anti-Semitism, which she believed to be a significant factor in the trajectory of Pappworth's career. Small, northern, Jewish: as a medical establishment outlier, Maurice Pappworth was in a prime position to criticise, expose and voice uncomfortable truths. As Bamber herself put it: 'He was a whistle-blower.'

Above all, Pappworth believed that ethics came first. Writing at a time when enthusiasm for science burned perhaps more strongly than it does in this more cynical age, he insisted that 'the pursuit of new scientific knowledge should not be allowed to take precedence over moral values where the two are in conflict'. These moral values, rooted in the principles of all our great religions, come back once again to the Golden Rule: 'Any human being has the right to be treated with a certain decency, and this right, which is individual, supersedes every consideration of what may benefit science or contribute to the public welfare.' I can still remember the shock I felt when, as a child watching my father on television, I heard him declare that it would be unjustifiable to find a cure for cancer if this meant 'killing a few people' along the way. Now, writing as someone who suffers from an incurable type of cancer, I can only agree with him.

Chapter One

From Lomza to Liverpool: a healer's hinterland

*'Certainly neither our parents nor we ourselves had any material pos-
sessions which could be called luxuries by any stretch of the imagination.'*

(from Maurice Pappworth's tape-recorded memoir)

In the Beginning

Maurice Pappworth was an outsider. He came from a family of outsiders, for
whom it took a generation as new immigrants before they could confidently
feely they truly belonged. Even then, there was certainly no shortage of occasions when they were reminded of their strangeness. He was a maverick doctor
who was unafraid to speak his mind. And it was partly because he felt treated
as an outsider that Maurice Pappworth had, apparently, so few qualms about
blowing the whistle on the British medical establishment.

His family story begins in the twelfth century, when Jews first settled in the
town of Lomza (pronounced 'Wodja'), north of Warsaw. Expelled in 1556, the
Jews were permitted by the Congress of Vienna in 1815 to return to Lomza
after an enforced absence of 260 years. From the mid-nineteenth century, Jews
played a prominent role in the economic life of Lomza, especially in the whole-
sale timber and grain trades. They involved themselves in the municipal administration until 1926, when a decree was issued forbidding Jews from this sphere.
They were also actively involved in the Polish uprisings of 1830, 1848 and
1863. Once Jews were cut off from work in local administration and found
themselves facing an impoverished life, many emigrated. It was also in 1926
that the Lomza Yeshiva (a place of Jewish learning) where Pappworth's grandfather and great grandfather studied, was closed down. It is a testament to the
Jewish determination to survive, culturally and intellectually, that in the very
year of its closure the Lomza Yeshiva reopened in Palestine, in Peta Tikvah.

Lomza has changed hugely since the Second World War. Its twenty-first
century approach takes visitors past roadside billboards reminiscent of some
town in the American mid-west. Through it flows the River Bug (pronounced

'Book'), within a wide valley. This river played its part in the story of the Pappworth emigration from Poland. Today, Lomza is a centre of the brewing industry, and the local beer is, apparently, much to be recommended. In the town centre some old buildings remain. Efforts are clearly being made to create a more attractive main square, which is flanked by houses painted in different colours and dotted with trees. It is still possible to walk through what was the Jewish ghetto. On its surprisingly wide main road, Senatorska Street, number 7 marks the old Jewish orphanage, which is still standing. Further down the street is the Jewish hospital, built in 1879 and now a school. A bronze plaque on the wall marks the edge of the ghetto: crowned by a Star of David, its commemoration is in Polish, and a bronze relief shows a group of anonymous faces – those for whom this town was once home.

Between the ghetto and the town square a ceramic relief features a Jewish cantor – known in Hebrew as a 'chazan' – and a Catholic pastor (among others), with explanations in Polish and English. The juxtaposition seems to suggest that, for many years, Jews and Christians lived in relative harmony. This was not, however, the experience of Maurice Pappworth's parents.

Reba Michal Ben Josef-Aron Luckl, a leading cantor in Lomza after 1918, was known for his strong baritone. He composed music for the prayers performed by the choir, which he conducted himself. 'He was kind to people,' runs the tribute, 'and followed God's word.' He was killed by the Germans in the Gielezynski Forest during the mass executions that took place in 1941. The Great Synagogue in Lomza, built between 1878 and 1899, included a famous rabbinic higher school run by Rabbi Eliezer Szulawicz. The synagogue was destroyed during the Second World War.

In those days the family name was Papperovitch, meaning 'the child of Papa'. The Russians had forced Jewish families to use the patronymic form for surnames. Jews create their surnames from their parents' first names – and these remain as what is known as one's 'Hebrew name', by which one is called up to participate in the synagogue service. So Maurice Henry Pappworth was Moshe Elkanan ben Yitzhak Yaakov ve Miriam Devorah, 'ben' meaning 'son', 've' meaning 'and'.

Samuel Hirsch Papperovitch, Maurice Pappworth's paternal great-grandfather, lived in Lomza with his wife, whom their great-grandson believed had the almost identical surname of Papparovitch. It is likely that they married in their teens. He was a Kest, meaning he spent more than forty years as a student and later a teacher in the Yeshiva, supported financially by his father-in-law. He was awarded a Biblical diploma, the Zomarha, and also managed to run a part-time timber business and a bakery – the latter organised and supervised by his wife. She died when her husband was in his sixties, at which point – after the mandatory year of mourning – Samuel Hirsch married a widow over thirty years his junior who already had three children. Her name was Esther, but she was always known as Spilker, which in Yiddish means 'plaything'.

Samuel's son and Maurice's paternal grandfather was Yisshur Chayim Papperovitch, born and brought up in Lomza. For several years his father taught him at the local Yeshiva where he studied. Although he had been a Kest, he was a businessman at heart, dealing, like his father, in timber, but also becoming involved in property refurbishment. He died in Poland in the early 1920s, over a hundred years old. In his seventies and possibly eighties he visited England and New York to see his emigrant offspring. Travelling by boat from Poland to Hamburg and then on to New York via Liverpool (where he stayed with his son, Maurice's father) and London must have been quite an undertaking. But the Papperovitch/Pappworth family have always described themselves as 'stoical', so Yisshur Chayim would have taken the journey in his stride.

Yisshur Chayim married Miriam Cohen, with whom he had five children. The eldest of these, Avram Tuvia, at the age of twenty-one, drowned in the local river. While he was swimming, so the family story goes, some Christian boys pelted him with stones and knocked him unconscious. The second child, Rosuria, who had three children, was murdered alongside two of them at a concentration camp in Poland – most probably Auschwitz, as it was to here that the Jews of Lomza were generally deported. Just one, Rachel, survived. In the 1920s she emigrated to the United States.

The third child was Yitzhak Yaakov, father of Maurice, who was followed by Hannah: her husband Elkanan Jepcovitz was conscripted into the Russian army for four years. On his release, he emigrated with Hannah to New York, changing his name to Henry Rosen. The youngest two were Etta, known as Maschitka, who got married in Liverpool but who doesn't appear to have maintained any contact with the family, and Sam, who developed a large dental practice in Brooklyn. When I visited my father's New York family in 1973, I met Sam Rosen and his wife Betty, and also their dentist son Bernard, all of whom lived on Long Island. But it was in Brooklyn that I stayed, with the eldest of Hannah and Henry's five children, Fanny Nagelberg.

Hannah's daughter, Minnie Dublin, was the one cousin with whom my father kept in regular touch, and she came to my sister Dinah's wedding in Jerusalem in 1980. She didn't have far to travel: when her husband died in the late 1960s, she decided to do that which, in her interpretation, is the thing God requires all Jews to do: return to the land of Zion which He gave to us. So this elderly woman said farewell to the life in Brooklyn she had always known, to her daughter Dorothy (a nurse) and son Bobby (a doctor), and to her seven grandchildren, and set off to live in an alien country which she saw as her true home. She settled in Dizengoff Avenue in Tel Aviv, a noisy thoroughfare, in a small flat where she lived until her death.

So we come to Yitzhak Yaakov/Isaac Jacob, the third of Yissur Chayim and Miriam Papperovitch's children, and Maurice Pappworth's father. My memories of him, with his full crop of thick straight white hair and white moustache, are of a benevolent old man bearing a strong resemblance to Father Christmas. But in his younger days this man, who was never seen out of doors without his top hat, ruled his family with a rod of iron, and seems to have given his six daughters a particularly hard time. His youngest, Naomi, in her unpublished *Chapters of an Autobiography*, recalls: 'My father was a dim presence who went to work early, came home late, had his meal and then sat by the fire smoking his pipe, disregarded except when a fierce outbreak of temper had him throwing himself between his fighting younger sons, lashing out in all directions, accompanied by a fine flow of Yiddish curses (favourites were something about being afflicted by a black year and "hang yourself and drown yourself") until mother intervened to save her young.' In her other work of family history, *Chronicles of the Papperovitch Family*, Naomi does admit that occasionally the atmosphere was relaxed, and her parents would play dominoes or draughts. 'This was a great treat… Once he sat me on his knee. I was very pleased.'

I remember as a small child being addressed by 'Grandad' (who was then in his eighties) as 'Wilder Chayah': an interesting Yiddish mixture of German and Hebrew meaning 'Wild Creature' (not a very appropriate moniker for the little girl I was). My sister Dinah was 'Chutzpah-Diknik'. In her *Chronicles*, Naomi observes that her father's education had been confined to the Hebrew Prayer Book. 'He could read only Hebrew characters. He never learned to write in any language. I once tried to teach him how to write his name, but he was an extremely bad, impatient pupil. As a result, when his signature was required we had to resort to forgery.'

When Naomi won a state scholarship to university, a form had to be signed by the parent and witnessed by a magistrate. Her eldest brother, Avram, obligingly forged their father's signature. 'I then took the document to one JP after another, all of whom said "I have not witnessed your father's signature, so I cannot sign." Finally, late at night, desperate that I would have to forgo my scholarship, I arrived at the house of the Mayor of Birkenhead. When he too refused his signature, I burst into hysterical sobs and he relented.'

Yitzhak had left Poland in search of a new life during the early 1880s. Maurice claimed that, among several reasons for his wanting to emigrate, one was his sadness at the tragic death by drowning of his elder brother Avram Tuvia. In a tape-recorded family history and autobiography, Maurice described Avram as his father's 'great and constant companion.' That this death was as a direct result of aggressive anti-Semitism will have provided Yitzhak with an additional incentive to turn his back on Poland forever.

There was also a strong probability that he would be conscripted into the Polish or Russian army for anything from four (like his brother-in-law Elkanan) to twenty-five years. According to Naomi, Yitzhak *was* in fact conscripted into the Tsar's army, hastening his decision to leave. He disliked the forced use of the patronymic Russian surname, and had no objection when in 1932 his eldest son, Avram David, changed his name by deed poll when called to the Bar. The whole family followed suit, their surname changing from Papperovitch to Pappworth. Maurice changed his by deed poll in 1933, when he embarked on his medical career. Why Avram David (A.D.) chose the double 'p' in the middle is unclear; indeed, Leah and Naomi, the two youngest daughters, always spelled it with just one 'p'.

So Yitzhak Yaakov Papperovitch put himself in the hands of an agent (possibly illegal, almost certainly charging extortionate rates) for the long boat trip to a better life. According to Naomi's *Chronicles*, Yitzhak did at one point before the First World War go off to America, leaving his wife behind in England with a brood of children. His niece Minnie, with whom Naomi kept in close touch, remembered him turning up at her mother's house in Brooklyn without warning, carrying a suitcase full of samples of English cloth with which he hoped to make his fortune. He later told Naomi that he had got as far west as St Louis, Missouri, before deciding that England would suit him better.

Certainly his initial emigration was straight to England, via Hamburg. He had in fact expected to sail to 'the Goldener Medina' of America, but instead found himself landing in east London. Here he was helped by a Jewish charity which met the boats at the docks and tried to find lodgings and jobs for the new immigrants. Yitzhak must have arrived hungry, exhausted and dishevelled. The boats did not contain bunks, so he would have brought his own bedding and slept on the floor of the deck. He would also have brought his own kosher food.

This may have been prepared for him by his new wife, Miriam Devorah from Ostrolenka. She was the daughter of Moshe Baruch Poplowicz, who was a Rebbe – someone who taught the rudiments of Hebrew prayer-reading to boys preparing for their barmitzvah. For this, according to Naomi, he was 'paid a pittance by their parents, who could hardly spare the few kopeks to pay him'. Miriam's mother had died young, at which point her thirteen-year-old daughter took over the running of the household. When her father re-married, Miriam grew to detest her stepmother, who treated her unkindly. As Ostrolenka and Lomza were more than twenty miles apart, it is likely that Yitzhak and Miriam's marriage was arranged by a broker – known as a Shadchan.

Miriam's new husband promised to make arrangements for her to join him in England once he was established. This took some time. He stayed in London for less than a year, working in a tailoring workshop in what amounted to sweatshop conditions. In Lomza, surrounded by extensive woodland, he had like his father and grandfather worked in timber. He probably became a tailor on his arrival in London chiefly because it seemed the most reliable means to employment.

Outsiders in Birkenhead

By the time Miriam emigrated from Poland to join her young husband, he had moved to Liverpool. They lived initially in the city's almost exclusively Jewish quarter, centred on the axis of Brownlow Hill, which comes up from Lime Street to the area now occupied by University buildings and the Roman Catholic Cathedral. The whole area was demolished during the Second World War. Now that he is in England, let us refer to Yitzhak as Isaac. He used his second name – Jacob – as the 'surname' of his business, opening a tailor's workshop where Miriam and later their eldest daughter, Hetty, worked. On the outbreak of the First World War in 1914, he won a contract to make khaki trousers for the army. His illiteracy did not seem to impede Isaac's conduct of business or everyday affairs. Naomi's theory was that 'he must have been very observant and had an excellent memory' – qualities inherited by both her and Maurice.

Within a few months of the outbreak of war, Isaac, Miriam and their now completed family of nine children moved to Birkenhead. There was in fact a tenth child, the second eldest. He died when still a small baby. Naomi noted in her *Chronicles* that 'He was never spoken of.' My father never mentioned to me the unknown older brother. Naomi maintains that the children were never told anything about their parents' harsh experiences. They occasionally spoke of "der haim" (the home), always in a tone of affection. To them, home was Russia, to which their part of Poland belonged, the country having been partitioned during the late eighteenth century between Russia, Prussia and Austria. The Papperovitches' hatred of anti-Semitic Poles meant that they did not communicate with their non-Jewish neighbours. They knew no Polish, except for a few words. Yiddish was their language.

'My mother's babies arrived at two-year intervals,' observes Naomi in her *Autobiography*, 'until Sidney was born only seventeen months after Maurice.' Born in June, Sidney was the only Papperovitch child who wasn't a winter baby. The family consisted of Hetty (born in 1896), Fanny, Rebecca (known always by Maurice as 'Rivkah' – her Hebrew name, and by Naomi as 'Becky'), Avram David (referred to by his siblings as 'A.D.' or 'Aby'), Esther, Leah, Maurice (born on 9 January 1910), Sidney (1911) and Naomi – who broke the two-yearly pattern by being born in December 1915. 'I heard my mother tell someone,' she recalls, 'that she had expected Sidney to be her last.' She cannot recall her parents sharing a bed.

As Naomi remembers it, her mother slept with Fanny after the latter became ill, her father with Sidney, Becky with Leah, Aby with Maurice and she herself with Esther. There was also always a cat attached to the family. 'Then one day,' Naomi tells us, 'Dad brought home a tiny black and white mongrel terrier puppy and gave him to me. I called him Jacky and lavished all my affection on him.' She used to sing to him, 'I will buy a licence for you if no-one else will pay. Jacky, oh Jacky, please do stay.' A licence then cost 7/6d a year. It reveals much about the emotional limitations of the Papperovitch family that Naomi found in her love for her dog an outlet for pent-up affections that could be channelled nowhere else. Jacky died at about sixteen, 'never having been taken to the vet and fed mainly on scraps, including all the bones from hens and fish which are now believed to be so harmful'.

On his father's decision to move the family across the Mersey from Liverpool, Maurice comments in the autobiography that he tape-recorded in the 1980s: 'Why he chose Birkenhead, which was then a town of only twenty to twenty-five Jewish families and has in fact never had more than that, I do not know. Perhaps the authenticated vandalism and harassment of foreigners, especially in the Jewish neighbourhood of Liverpool, was a determining factor.' Naomi was similarly puzzled, especially by their father's choice of neighbourhood within Birkenhead: 'It was far away from the shopping centre of the town and, there being no Jews within miles, it was, in my mother's words, "Farvarfen from Menschen"' – far away from people. According to Naomi, 'we were known in the neighbourhood as "the Jews." This was in no way pejorative. They were not anti-Semitic. We were the only Jews for miles around, so it was simply a statement of fact.'

The family settled at first into number 15 Greenway Road, but within less than a year moved to number 5, a combined house and shop. In Naomi's *Chronicles of the Papperovitch Family* number 5 'was the villain of the family story. I was sure that it had a malevolent influence on our lives… It was a horrible house… Greenway Road ran along the top of a low ridge, where had once stood the hamlet of Higher Tranmere. A few eighteenth-century cottages still survived: halfway up the road, with the long, narrow front gardens common in villages… they had degenerated into a slum, inhabited by ragged bare-foot children and foul-mouthed adults.'

The shop had its own entrance and a large display window, where Isaac showed off a few lengths of cloth. Number 3 Greenway Road was also a shop, 'a sweet shop, tobacconist, newsagent and post office,' according to Maurice. Naomi recalls that this belonged to a childless couple called Bishop, who were 'fascinated by the goings-on of the huge foreign family next door.' Between the Bishop and Papperovitch shops was a high walled passage about six feet wide.

Maurice remembers two large high cellars, the one under the shop being used to store coal. Also in this cellar was a narrow room with a shelf and a bench which Maurice's older brother Avram David, and later Maurice himself, used as a photographic dark room. This was to become the start of a lifelong passion for taking, developing and printing his own photographs. The other cellar, below the main part of the house, was equipped with a copper boiler and a small oven, used for 'the large weekly laundry, which my mother did usually all on her own.' Nearby stood a large metal washtub with scrubbing board and a mangle – manually operated, of course. I find myself wondering in awe at this life of the Rebbe's daughter, labouring in a dark cellar in a foreign land for a family of eleven over washtub and mangle.

Naomi's remembers that, in the cellar, 'every Monday, my mother spent the whole day doing the family wash. She was a tiny woman: less than five feet tall, dressed in an old skirt and blouse, several aprons tied round her waist to keep out the wet, her arms and hands rough and red from constant immersion in water. Her face never knew any cosmetics; her hair was screwed... tight into a little bun at the back of her head. Not until she had it cut short (to make it easier to cope with when she was ill), did one realise what pretty silky, fine, naturally wavy hair it was. Then one remembered the story of my father seeing her long dark hair for the first time before their wedding. He said that it was too beautiful to be cut off to make way for the customary sheitel [wig worn by orthodox Jewish women], which she never wore.'

'In my memory,' Naomi continues, 'she is bent double over a huge wooden tub, scrubbing dirty clothes on a washboard, or using tremendous energy to manipulate a wooden "dolly" in a zinc barrel-shaped tub... Finally, she hung the clothes either on lines across the cellar or, in fine weather, in the yard. In the midst of this exhausting work she found time to cook a large mid-day dinner for her children. She emerged into the kitchen, smelling of wash day, to serve us soup, meat and potatoes. She never sat down with us. I don't know when and where she herself ate. We accepted what she gave us. No-one offered to help. No-one suggested she might be exhausted.'

Naomi writes that 'I used to follow her about the house, often clinging to her long skirts. I was afraid to be alone. I don't remember that we ever talked to each other or that she helped me in any way to play. She never caressed any of her children or gave any outward sign of affection. When she came to see me in hospital after I, a ten-year-old, had my appendix out, she hugged and kissed me. It astonished me so much I was embarrassed.'

It is hardly surprising that, with this constant round of domestic chores, Miriam did not have time to be a mother in other, less tangible ways. Naomi recalls that she was 'always too busy, cooking and washing and shopping, to talk to me, and kissing and cuddling was not in her nature'. The Papperovitch siblings remained, throughout their lives, wary of demonstrating physical affection. Kissing continued to be an awkward ritual, clearly not enjoyed.

'On Shabbas [Friday night preceding the Sabbath] there was always chicken,' Naomi recalls – 'or rather, hen. Mother bought this live at a market in Liverpool and brought it home in a large straw bag. It was then released into the back yard until it could be taken across Birkenhead to Rebbe Finkelstein's house to be ritually slaughtered. This was usually Esther's job, which she hated.

Once mother was badly pecked by an angry hen and had a poisoned hand.' The hen was made into rich chicken soup. Maurice, in his recorded memoir, remembers his mother making the *lockshen* (vermicelli) for the Sabbath chicken soup. 'On Friday night we very rarely had any other meal than chicken soup and lokshen with either roast or boiled chicken as a first course, followed by a lokshen or other pudding as a sweet.'

Maurice also admired the way his mother, for every Shabbat or festival, made a challah (the Jewish plaited loaf containing egg). She had an arrangement with Mr Turtle, who ran the bakery across from their house in Greenway Road, whereby she carried the tins containing the loaves she had made over the road and Mr Turtle would put them into an oven using a long pole. According to Naomi, their mother didn't buy the family's everyday bread (of which they ate huge quantities) from Turtle's but from the Co-op, because the latter 'gave "divi" – a few coppers for every pound spent. 'That divi played an important part in Mother's housekeeping.'

Not only did Miriam rarely sit down with her family to eat a meal: she also deprived herself of social contacts outside the home. She seldom went out, except to shop for food. Once a week she visited the Jewish shops on Brownlow Hill, Liverpool, to buy kosher meat, pickled cucumbers, pickled or salted herrings and *schmaltz* (chicken fat) selected from barrels. Back home, Miriam made the meat fully kosher by salting it herself. She also fried huge quantities of fish for the family, and the habit of eating cold fried fish for several days in a row was passed on to the next generation when, years later, Esther taught my mother the recipe.

Maurice calls his mother 'a genuine *ayshet chayil*' – a 'woman of worth,' as described in the Book of Proverbs: 'a woman of courage, devotion and resourcefulness. She was a Yiddish momma in the original and genuine meaning of that term, namely a Jewish woman who was prepared to spend her life in the service of God and devotion to her husband and children, always putting their interests and needs before her own.' Without much help from her children, Maurice's mother gave the whole house its statutory spring clean immediately prior to Passover, all traces of *chometz* (leavened foods) being removed and cutlery boiled to destroy any contamination by leavening agents. A special set of crockery is kept for use only during the eight days of Passover: this practice must have strained Isaac's finances. The food was delivered by the kosher grocery.

Maurice did not find in his wife the martyr he admired in his mother, and my recollections of Passover are of my father doing the cleaning and preparation himself, rushing around the kitchen with pans of boiling water while we unwrapped the special festival china. Meanwhile my mother lay awake for a fortnight before Seder night (the festive meal that marks the start of Passover), worrying how she was going to cook dinner for fifteen to twenty people when she wasn't allowed to start work on it until everything was *Pesach-dikker* (kosher for Passover) – a goal rarely achieved before mid-to-late afternoon on the day of the feast.

A Merseyside childhood

Maurice in his recorded memoir chooses to convey a more positive image of 5 Greenway Road. Whereas Naomi recalls that steps from the cellar led to the 'back yard', he prefers to refer to this plot as a 'small garden,' consisting of 'a rockery with a single lilac tree'. At the back of the garden was a midden – a hole in the wall with an iron door on the garden side and another on the outside, which led out onto an alleyway known on Merseyside as a 'jigger.' The whole of the rear of the garden was covered by a flat wooden structure supported by the stone wall of the midden, with a beam running along its roof from which hung two large metal hoops. 'From that,' Maurice tells us, 'we children dangled ropes connected at the end with a plank used as a seat and the whole contraption became a swing, on which certainly myself, Sidney and Naomi [the three youngest children] enjoyed many happy moments.' Naomi makes no mention of the swing.

The rest of the house was, according to Maurice, on three floors. 'A few wooden stairs led through a door, almost always locked, from the shop itself into a parlour,' Maurice recalls. 'The only thing that I remember about that parlour was that it contained a large round table always covered with a cloth. This was the room where visitors not considered to be of so-called importance were usually entertained.' The Papperovitches were not keen entertainers. Naomi, in *Chapters of an Autobiography*, notes that her school-friends 'had lovely parties and did not seem to mind that I never invited them back home.' She adds: 'We Papperovitches never went on holiday, but when, at the beginning of the autumn term, we were asked to write about "The happiest day of my holiday", I had no difficulty in improvising.' The school holidays could none-theless be enjoyable. Greenway Road at that time was on the edge of town, and Naomi recalls going for long country walks.

But the house was a frightening place. The two youngest children in partic-ular were frightened of its dark cellar, 'peopled,' in Naomi's imagination, 'by undesirable horrors'. It is hardly surprising that, for Maurice, to live in a sub-stantial house in a desirable area was one of his chief ambitions. Naomi com-ments in her *Chronicles*, 'As I sit now in great comfort in my well-equipped Highgate flat, I almost disbelieve in that other me in that squalid house... Yes, I remember, I remember the house where I was born, and the memory is still hateful to me.'

Maurice never openly stated such a negative attitude, but there can be no doubt that his childhood home was a chief impetus in his determination to pros-per. This is probably something his wife Jean, raised in affluence, never entirely understood. In his taped autobiography, Maurice says that he has 'no means of knowing' how successful his father's business was, 'and perhaps it is best summed up by a favourite saying of his: "I make a living." We were at least as well fed and clothed as any other children in the neighbourhood, which was essentially... middle class... Certainly neither our parents nor we ourselves had any material possessions which could be called luxuries by any stretch of the imagination.'

Often, on a Sunday, Maurice or Sidney was allowed to accompany the local dairy-owner Mr Johnson on his rounds in a pony-drawn cart. A related memory of Maurice's is of the cows kept in a shed in a side road off Brownlow Hill, which never went out to grass. Their milk was sold to the Orthodox Jews of the neighbourhood, with the guarantee that that it had not been touched by non-Jews. Maurice comments: 'It was very unlikely that that milk was ever pasteur-ised, and it was probably the enactment of a law making pasteurisation com-pulsory which led to the abandonment of keeping milking cows in sheds in cities.' At the end of Greenway Road was 'a genuine dairy farm,' where at Passover time the Papperovitchs took jugs to be filled directly from the cows, thus ensuring that the milk was free of the forbidden 'chometz' (leavening).

On their way to the farm the children would gaze up at the most prominent local landmark – a water tower. During the First World War, they walked past allotments and, as they descended the hill, uncultivated grass fields. 'Later, over this area... a housing estate was built, of pebble-dash, semi-detached houses with small gardens in front and rear, which were occupied by middle-class professional people…' The roads were named after Birkenhead climbers George Mallory and Sandy Irvine, who lost their lives in 1924 on Everest. Not all the fields were built over. Some later became the playing fields for Birkenhead Institute, the secondary school attended by the three Papperovitch boys – Avram, Maurice and Sidney.

These playing fields represented another of Maurice's great enthusiasms: sport. In his recorded account, one can sense the breathless thrill for a boy just starting out at a new school. 'There were two full-sized football pitches and, in the central area, a cricket pitch between them.' A street or two away lay the grounds of Tranmere Rovers Football Club. 'The secretary of Tranmere Rovers often allowed Sidney and myself to watch matches free of charge. My father regarded that as "non-Jewish nonsense", which was a favourite remark of his. He allowed us to do so because we did not break Shabbat law by conducting any financial transaction, namely the payment of the entrance fee.'

Their father seems to have had a strict but not entirely consistent attitude to Jewish observance. Naomi remembered him going out to work at his tailoring business on the Sabbath, but also – all too clearly – his response when, after her first Christmas at school, she 'came home and told the lovely story of the baby born in a manger. My father was furious. I was forbidden ever to mention this again. The school was told that I must never go to Scripture lessons.' But conversations with the nine siblings during my own childhood revealed not a single joyous memory of times spent as a family on Shabbat (the Sabbath) or at any of the Jewish festivals. Although the boys went through barmitzvah, it seems that only their father attended synagogue to witness the ceremony; there was no celebration at home afterwards. When she started at Birkenhead High School, having been awarded a scholarship, Naomi felt different from the other girls not so much from inequality of family wealth, but because of her Jewishness – 'the only Jewish girl who had ever been a pupil at B.H.S…. On my very first day I was confronted by Phyllis Tame, daughter of the Town Clerk, with the words "You killed Christ."' The art teacher was openly anti-Semitic. It is perhaps not so surprising that Maurice felt haunted throughout his career by the demon of anti-Jewish sentiment.

Of all the Papperovitch children, Maurice was the most committed to his Judaism. His verdict on being exempted by his grammar-school headmaster from morning prayers, and from lessons on Saturday mornings and Jewish festivals, was 'I am confident that missing school on a Saturday morning had no serious effect on our [his, A.D.'s and Sidney's] education.... I was always in the top grade.' (As a child, I deeply resented the way our father insisted we miss school for every Jewish festival, and could not share his complacency about these enforced absences' lack of impact.) As a boy he went to a small group who took Hebrew instruction from the Reverend Finkelstein (the 'Rebbe' Naomi mentions who doubled up as the ritual slaughterer, or Shochet).

Maurice decided to continue his Jewish education for another two years after his barmitzvah. His youthful immersion in Jewish philosophy and ethics was to have a profound influence on his attitude to the treatment of patients, and to medical issues in general. Maurice was a great admirer of Reverend Finkelstein, whose deep knowledge extended across a range of areas both intellectual and practical, from classical and modern Hebrew to Jewish religion and philosophy. 'An interesting point was that he certainly was not recognised, or in any way appreciated, by members of the congregation.' Maurice Pappworth attached importance to the recognition of high quality in people, whatever their profession.

Greenway Road eventually became Bebington Road, leading to Bebington, Port Sunlight and the main roads to Chester and the western part of the Wirral. Nearby, Victoria Park offered lawns, flowers and – of more interest to Maurice and Sidney – tennis courts and a rolled lawn for bowls. 'From the road immediately outside the park railings... a steep descent allowed a splendid view of Camel Laird's ship-building yard, with the berthed ships visible on a fine day and the prominent buildings on the Liverpool side of the Mersey.'

On the southern side of Birkenhead, extending towards Rock Ferry, was Mersey Park, where, as a teenager, Maurice played cricket in the evening, 'before or after doing my homework.' In the northern part of town lay the largest of its public parks, Birkenhead Park. This boasted tropical and semi-tropical greenhouses, an artificial boating lake, tennis courts, football pitches and 'cricket pitches with pavilions.' During the summer, 'I often walked by myself for two or three miles each day to watch the cricket match while sitting on the grass verge.'

The only negative aspect to this idyllic memory is that the Birkenhead Cricket Club's members came mostly from fee-paying Birkenhead School, 'considered to be the snobbish equivalent of the grammar school which I attended, and ... preferred by the wealthier families'. Nevertheless, the Birkenhead Institute had its moments on this sacred ground: 'my grammar school team, of whom I was a member when in the upper forms, played each Wednesday afternoon.' The only clear memory Maurice records from his earlier, elementary school days is a sporting one: he arrived in the middle of a cricket match against a rival school and, his team being one short, he was brought on to make up the eleven. 'I was in fact the top scorer but unfortunately my school lost.' Later, he regularly played cricket and (as a right half) football.

Not once does Maurice mention that, as a small child, he suffered from rickets. This illness does not appear to have had a significant physical impact on him, however, apart from his small stature: he was about five feet four inches tall and remained slim all his life. Indeed, pictures of him as a young man (he had a large collection) show someone proud of his athletic physique and his fair-haired good looks. He was also physically affected at the age of about eight by an unpleasant experience: walking home from school, he was suddenly set upon by boys who fired peashooters at him. Judging by photographs of him and Sidney at this age, the two brothers still had their hair in long ringlets. It has been suggested that the attackers were schoolfellows mocking his effeminate hairstyle.

Dodging out of their range, Maurice darted into the road, only to be knocked down by a horse-drawn cab. He 'was found to be badly bruised and had a large cut on my chin, the scar of which persists to this day'. I remember that scar. As always, the Papperovitch parents seem to have been very relaxed about their child's well-being.

In 1926, when she was ten, Naomi spent a weekend vomiting. Yet she was sent to school on the Monday, 'But when I kept on vomiting there, I was sent home alone. When I came into the kitchen, mother was frying fish on the fire. I said, "Mother, I've been sent home. I've been sick." She did not turn around to look at me. She went on frying fish and said, "Have a drink of water." That night it became obvious to everybody that I really was ill. Dr Temple arrived, pronounced that I had acute appendicitis and must be sent, by ambulance, to the Children's Hospital. Mother would not allow this because some of the doctors there were women. So, after an argument and delay, I ended up as the only child in an adult ward in the local infirmary, where I was operated on by a surgeon who, soon afterwards, was dismissed for being drunk on the job.'

The picture Maurice paints of his Birkenhead years in his taped memoir is an attractive, even affectionate one. Perhaps, as some people do in their memoirs, his chooses to turn his back on the less pleasant aspects of childhood.

These are sketched in much darker colours in his younger sister Naomi's recollections. One is left wondering whether it was purely professional ambition that made Maurice so determined to move away from Merseyside – or whether he found growing up and going to university there more difficult than he was prepared to admit.

After the First World War, Isaac let the shop in Greenway Road to a demobilised solder, a cobbler called Mr Jones. As the result of a shell wound, Jones had an artificial leg. 'He often allowed me to watch him at work,' records Maurice, 'and I still vividly remember the selection of different sized sold metal lasts on which the shoe repairs were fitted. I also remember the large sheets of leather, from which he skilfully cut the heels and soles with a very large curved knife. I also remember the machine for sewing the leather but, best of all, I recall how he filled his mouth with small metal nails which he extracted from his mouth one by one and hammered each into the new soles and heels.' Maurice always prided himself on his memory and Mr Jones, with his mouth full of nails, does have the vividness of a permanently stamped impression. Throughout his life, he respected the skills of others, whether a car mechanic, a pianist, an electrician or a cook. Brought up 'above the shop,' watching his mother work punishing hours on household chores and his sisters busy all day at sewing machines in the workshop, surrounded by neighbours who worked long hours at their trade or profession, he was intolerant of idleness.

Isaac then rented a large workshop in Cable Street, Liverpool. In both Liverpool and Birkenhead, he traded under the name of 'Jacobs' – doubtless more palatable than 'Papperovitch' to his English customers. Most of the labour was female. From among his six daughters, Hetty was later joined by Esther. The women were principally seamstresses, sewing by hand and machine. At least one was also employed to do the ironing. The solid irons weighed over ten pounds each; these were heated on heavy gas burners. 'My father himself was the cutter,' recalls Maurice, 'who chalked on the cloth the outline of the garment and then cut it accordingly.' He also assisted with the ironing. The number of his employees depended on the time of year, varying from six to about fourteen. And so, in his own words, he managed to 'make a living'.

With the economic slump of the 1920s at its height, believing that the recession would not last long and would swiftly be followed by a boom, Isaac made a decision 'probably on bad advice from one of his cronies'. He disposed of his pedal-operated sewing machines and bought a set of the latest electric versions. But the promised recovery did not materialise. Isaac had to abandon the Cable Street workshop – though he didn't find himself bankrupt. Some of the machines were stored in a shed belonging to a furniture remover near the Greenway Road house. Isaac's eldest son, A.D., by now a graduate in his twenties, resented his father's stubbornly uncommunicative stance: his plans for the business were never discussed. But Maurice remembered 'overhearing conversations between my father and my mother about those machines… My father, always being optimistic, believed he would one day make good use of them.'

The event was a turning point in the working life of Isaac Jacob. He eventually decided to re-occupy the shop in Greenway Road. His work there would consist, he hoped, in custom from neighbours and from the owners of tailoring shops in Birkenhead who sold made-to-measure suits but never made the garments themselves. Isaac planned to become one of those outside tailors to whom this work would be contracted. For several years one of the most successful tailors in Birkenhead, Armstrong's, gave him such work, but it was unsettlingly seasonal.

Now it was time for A.D. to step in. Entirely on his initiative and using his own money, he purchased for £600 number 29 Rocky Bank Road, in respectable middle-class Devonshire Park. The house was for his parents and the four siblings still living at home as well as for himself; he was to carry on living there for well over forty years. The family moved there in 1932. Maurice would have been twenty-two, and studying at Liverpool University. Hunched on the corner of the street, this house is still a rather forbidding edifice, a dark, moored hulk, and the final vessel of one family's voyage towards Englishness.

The Making of a Medic

At what stage Maurice Pappworth decided to train as a doctor is unclear. With an older brother forging a successful career as a lawyer, it perhaps seemed natural that, in this aspirational Jewish family, son number two (and, in the event, number three as well) should enter the medical profession. Pappworth's subsequent journey showed that, although he didn't choose to tread an easy path, he embarked, aged just sixteen, on a career at which he turned out to be a brilliant practitioner.

Having taken nine school subjects for matriculation, the maximum allowed, he worked on his three subjects for the Higher School Certificate. Of these, his favourite was chemistry. When, aged thirteen, I was struggling at school with chemistry, Dad gave me just a couple of lessons – and the proverbial scales fell from my eyes. Suddenly, I understood it. Maurice, in his taped memoir, included a story about his school experiences with chemistry. About one month before the exam, 'I was doing an experiment to attempt to find out the contents of a powder… The difficulty was that the substance had to be first dissolved and the only way that I could find to dissolve it was to add sulphuric acid. But when I added that substance to differentiate between the groups in this set of compounds, there was a minor explosion and the acid burst out onto my face. I was rushed to a doctor who lived a hundred yards from the school. I was extremely fortunate… but I remember I had to wear a mask covered with ointment for several weeks, and had only started to really recover when …the examination took place. Surprisingly my best subject then in the exam was chemistry, in which I got a distinction… The scars of that accident are still with me, and on my forehead I have emblazoned a letter M.'

As a child I believed him when he told me that the first letter of his name had been deliberately created with the help of acid. Bearing in mind his penchant for story-telling, it is difficult sometimes to assess how much of his taped autobiography is reliable. He always had an excellent memory, which stayed with him to the end, but from the days when he terrified his youngest sister with his bedtime stories, he enjoyed spinning a good yarn. The white scar on his forehead was quite prominent, and the co-incidental 'M' equally striking.

As a result of his marks for the Higher School Certificate, Maurice was awarded the school's Tate Scholarship to Liverpool University. This paid his fees and gave him a maintenance allowance of £20 a year (a third of the value of Naomi's later Oxford scholarship). His first year curriculum when he started at Liverpool University's Medical School in 1926 would have included biology (including zoology and botany), physics and chemistry, with a First MB exam in the Lent term. Anatomy and physiology then followed, to be continued into the second year, and examined in the summer term. The third year introduced students to *materia medica* and pharmacy, and to subjects ranging from bacteriology and general pathology to practical surgery, vaccination and clinical work. The fourth year culminated in the Final MB exam Part A. Systematic surgery, and clinical obstetrics or gynaecology, were also studied at this point, but not examined until the end of the fifth year, when studies included midwifery, infectious, mental and children's diseases, and opthalmology. The last three years of the five-year course were spent on clinical work in hospitals.

Determined to save money, Pappworth went home almost every day for lunch, during his first two years at least. Equally committed to Jewish doctrine, he never attended Saturday morning lectures. He managed, nevertheless, to be involved in sport and social life, and his active participation in the university's medical society struck a direct blow to the academic accolades he was so keen to win. He tells the story in his taped memoir: 'We had a medical students' society, and when I was in my fourth year students from the Faculty of Arts, both male and female, were invited to take part in a debate with us. The subject selected was, surprisingly and peculiarly, "Love is the greatest thing in life". I spoke, and said that the alternatives to love were mentioned in a recent novel…by [Leon] Feuchtwanger, and advised the audience to read that book and find the answers. But behind me was sitting one Joe Sitner, who was in his final year. He was a huge-sized chap, and very popular and witty. He later became a very successful GP in the less salubrious areas of Liverpool, and played a very active part as a Labour councillor. I had initially had no intention whatsoever on enlarging on that quote from Feuchtwanger. But Sitner, sitting behind me, in a very loud voice kept egging me on to do so, and very foolishly I did. Professor Hay was at that time in the Chair. I then mentioned that in the opinion of Feuchtwanger, the greatest things in life were eating, drinking, micturition, defecation and sex. Professor Hay immediately called on the next speaker.'

He continues: 'The following day the student President, Kenneth Bowes, who later became a Professor of Obstetrics at St Thomas' Hospital, London, insisted that I apologise both to him and also, in person, to Professor Hay. This I did. Years later, after Hay retired as Professor of Clinical Medicine at Liverpool, I got to know him personally much better, because I privately coached his two sons… He informed me at that time that he never forgot or forgave those remarks of mine at that debate, and although I was the best student in clinical medicine at the final examinations… he opposed giving me a distinction in clinical medicine, and I would have been the only one to have got such a distinction.'

This passage is so revealing of the man – not only his tendency to indulge in coarse humour, but also his subsequent regret, his excellence as a clinician, and the fact that, whatever fellow doctors thought of him personally, they were still keen to call on his medical and teaching expertise. It is an excellent instance of the way in which Pappworth took risks, often at some cost to himself. Times change, of course, and when, during the much more liberal 1960s and 1970s, Pappworth was invited to address students at the Liverpool Medical Students' Society, he was 'amazed, and perhaps even disgusted, at the sheer vulgarity and the frequent use of four-letter words and innuendos'. Even in this, it appears, he had been a trail-blazer.

During 1926-1927, Pappworth's first year, there were forty students in Liverpool Medical School's new intake. In his second year, the university's records show thirty-one men and just five women. Overall, students at the School in that year totalled 209. Among a list of extremely English names (it was to be several more years before he became 'Pappworth'), M.H. Papperovitch stands out with the Robert Gee prize in Paediatrics and the *proxime accessit* (runner-up) for the Gold Medal in Medicine. In his first year exams he was one of only six students (out of thirty-six) to gain a 1 in chemistry, and one of only four to gain a 1 in zoology. In botany, however, he was 'unclassified.' In December 1929 he passed his Second MB Part B and Third BDS Part A with 61 per cent. He gained a 1 in *materia medica*, but in practical pharmacy scored only a 3. However ambitious he may have been for stellar results (as a father he was rigorously so on his children's behalf), Pappworth clearly put his energies chiefly into what interested him. In July 1932 he graduated as M.B. CH.B (Hons.), with distinctions in Physics, Pharmacology and Therapeutics, and Obstetrics and Gynaecology.

Later, in April 1936, Pappworth was proud to be awarded his Membership of the Royal College of Physicians (MRCP) at the first attempt, without having attended any special tutorial classes, or resorted to private coaching. The exam had always had a notoriously high failure rate. In recognition of Pappworth's achievement, Liverpool awarded him a Samuel Scholarship of £50 for the best postgraduate student of the year. In December 1937, aged not quite twenty-eight, he gained his MD by examination, with Cardiology as a special subject.

While he was at Liverpool University, staff at all medical schools in the UK were encouraged to sign a petition to the House of Commons requesting that it should 'not support any bill which has for its object further restrictions upon experimental work on dogs or other animals'. This petition reminds us that there were strict laws governing animal experimentation in the UK – stricter than any that related to research on humans. It also draws attention to the vigilance of the medical profession in protecting its right to conduct research unimpeded. This attitude was to have a significant effect on the response to *Human Guinea Pigs*. For eighteen months, however, Pappworth himself was a part-time member of staff at the Liverpool Cancer Research Organisation, for which he performed routine biomedical and pharmacological work, testing on cats the toxicity of various lead preparations and on humans a modified Vernes serological test for cancer. As a young doctor, Pappworth doubtless felt that such experience was needed for his *curriculum vitae*.

Chapter Two

Roots and branches: a family in search of home

'Esther exclaimed in astonishment, "Whatever happened to you? You look as though you are going to explode." And that was how I felt. I had a light inside me.'

(from Naomi Pappworth's 'Chapters of Autobiography', recalling her high-school scholarship)

Hetty and Fanny: 'We are forbidden to cry on the Sabbath'

Hetty

The experiences of his brothers and sisters will help to explain more fully the influences that shaped Maurice Pappworth. Hetty, the eldest, was thirteen years his senior. It was she who worked at their father's workshop, having left school at fourteen so that she could help with the family business and look after the growing brood of younger siblings. After attending evening classes at the Workers' Educational Association, she was awarded a scholarship to Ruskin College, Oxford, at the time controlled by the trades unions and not part of Oxford University. Hetty seems to have been a restless young woman, who left Ruskin after less than a year, made a brief return to Birkenhead, and then went down to London to work as a housekeeper in Kensington until the outbreak of the Second World War. Naomi remembers her as very generous, and the source of treats when she came home to visit. 'On one visit she brought a young man and announced that they were engaged. I don't know what happened, but she never married.'

Hetty's next move was to Bournemouth, where she was in charge of a home for young male Jewish refugees from Europe. But her family did not know her address. When, after the war, Esther went to work for the Jewish Welfare Board, she often visited the Board's Home in Bournemouth. According to Naomi, 'She was told that someone of her name was living in poor circumstances. She went to visit and found Hetty crippled with rheumatoid arthritis.' She was living in a large neglected house in which she had been renting out rooms.

Eventually bed-ridden, she developed a chest infection. Esther was able to arrange for her sister to be admitted to the Jewish Welfare Board's Home for the Disabled. The matron, realising that Hetty's condition was rather more serious than the 'indigestion' for which she had for years been taking Digestive Rennies, had her transferred to a branch of St Thomas' Hospital in Surrey, where she remained until she died on 27 March 1956, aged fifty-nine. 'She was very brave,' recalls Naomi, 'and never complained of pain. She had a beautiful, unlined complexion and thick black hair to the end.' Naomi's diagnosis of her sister's final illness, unconfirmed by Maurice, was bowel cancer. 'When she actually did die,' continues Naomi, 'we did not tell my father and he never inquired after her. I don't know why we spared him.'

Fanny

Fanny, born at the turn of the century, was known affectionately as 'Feigele', meaning 'little bird'. Judging by photographs, she was very attractive, with auburn hair and blue/grey eyes. According to Naomi, she was tall for a Papperovitch. Fanny won a scholarship to pioneering Oulton Grammar School, which admitted pupils of both sexes. Fanny proceeded to teacher training college in Liverpool. But before she completed her diploma she developed ulcerative colitis – another disorder which seems to lurk in the Papperovitch genes – from which she never recovered. She was too ill to work. As Maurice explains: 'never having been employed, she was not eligible to be a panel patient, in the Lloyd George terminology before the National Health Service.' All doctors' visits and medicines had to be paid for. Watching Fanny suffer, and noting what he saw as the inadequacies of her medical care, will have made Maurice particularly conscious of the rights of patients. 'What I cannot understand,' he declares, 'is why, during the many years she was afflicted with this terrible disease, her GP never once sent her to be seen in a Liverpool teaching hospital, or even sent her to be an inpatient in a hospital, to be thoroughly investigated... Ever since I myself was qualified I have been puzzled by this serious omission.'

Like her older sister, Fanny developed rheumatoid arthritis, making any mobility impossible. The more immobile Fanny became, the fewer the friends who came to visit. 'So she sat by the bedroom fire,' recalls Naomi, 'or was pushed in the old-fashioned heavy bath-chair, usually by Becky, up to Victoria Park at the top of the road... She liked being read to, again usually by Becky.

But quite often I took a turn... except when Fanny decided that the book contained things too adult for my ears and I was not allowed to continue.'

Then Fanny was diagnosed with tuberculosis. 'It was only then,' recalls Maurice, 'that Dr Swan called in a senior physician from Liverpool Royal Infirmary... Dr Coupe [the senior physician looking after Fanny] told me he had been to see my sister, and expressed an opinion that the outlook was extremely grave and hopeless... This was before the days of antibiotics or any effective anti-tuberculosis chemotherapy. I well recall that he described Fanny as a very brave woman.' In Naomi's account, Becky brought along her old classmate Reggie Jones, who was to become the famous orthopaedic surgeon, Sir Reginald Watson-Jones. Naomi wondered whether he was doing his best to effect an improvement in her sister, 'Or was he treating Fanny as a guinea pig? By this time, she was completely bent over. He tried to straighten her spine. The treatment was horrific. He invented a frame of steel and leather on which she lay. It came up to her neck. There was a band to tie around her forehead, from which hung weights, to be increased in size as the treatment took effect. Then she went into hospital to be operated on; she came out in a worse state than ever. [Jones] had also tried to release her jaw – disastrously: her mouth was permanently twisted into a grimace, so that she did not even have the consolation of her good looks. After that, she gave up completely.' Awareness of what his sister was submitted to as a 'guinea pig' will have stalked the memory of the man who, thirty-eight years later, incorporated the phrase into the title of his book.

Fanny died in 1929, aged just thirty. Naomi, writing her family *Chronicles*, remembers the moment when she and Sidney, downstairs in the kitchen, 'heard one small cry. We knew that the end had come. It was a Friday in summer. My father came home, sat at the table, and mother gave him his dinner. Nothing was said. I don't know when he was told that his daughter had died. It was a normal Saturday, with the usual activities and no display of emotion. Then the day ended. It was dark. Mother gave out an enormous cry and broke into loud sobs. Next day when asked how it was that she had, for so long, controlled her grief, she answered, "Shabbas, torme nicht vainen" – "We are forbidden to cry on the Sabbath."' Fanny's illness, and the physical contact between them, resulted in Miriam's death from tuberculosis six years later.

Rivkah and A.D.: 'the martyrdom complex'

Rebecca, born in 1901, was known until middle age as 'Becky', but Maurice always called her by her Hebrew name, Rivkah. She appears to have been a significant influence on the lives of the three youngest children of the family. Throughout her life she remained close to Sidney, ten years her junior. Naomi, the youngest, recalls that when she was a child Becky was 'always jolly, affectionate and very kind to me. I cared far more for her than any of my siblings or my parents, who seemed remote, unresponsive and were far too busy to play.'

For Naomi, this sister was 'the most important person in my life… It was she who usually saw me to bed, where she recited poetry to me: [Robert Louis] Stevenson's *A Child's Garden of Verses* and Walter de la Mare's *Peach Pie* were favourites.' It was Becky who took her to the Walker Art Gallery and the Liverpool Museum. Naomi preferred it when Becky treated her to a show at the Liverpool Playhouse, where they paid sixpence and watched the performance from wooden benches at the back of the gallery. Becky also took her to see several plays by Bernard Shaw: 'I saw Sybil Thorndike as the original "St Joan" – I still remember it clearly.'

Rebecca was helping her younger siblings in their transition from the Eastern European, Yiddish culture of their parents to the British culture which she had already grown to love. She taught poetry to Maurice as well: in his sixties he was passing it on to me as I followed in my late aunt's footsteps and studied English at university. When I told my father I was studying Milton, he started to intone from *Comus*: 'Sabrina fair, listen where thou art sitting/ Under the glassy, cool, translucent wave…'

It was clear that Maurice had loved 'Rivkah' when he was a child and evidently a source of some sadness to him that, living so much closer to Sidney's family than to his, she grew very fond of the former's children but scarcely knew the three daughters of whom Maurice was so proud. In 1965 we went to visit her and A.D. in Birkenhead. My father, who was good at planning trips, made it part of a holiday that also took in the Cotswolds, North Wales and Shropshire. My eleven-year-old's impression of my eldest surviving aunt was of a tiny, highly excitable woman who rushed around, talking very fast, and who didn't seem quite sure how to relate to these three small daughters of the brother who had been so attached to her when he was their age.

Like Fanny, Rebecca won a scholarship to Oulton Grammar School, where she prospered. She was thought to be 'brilliant', according to Naomi, and was popular with pupils and teachers alike. In her Higher School Certificate (the more demanding precursor of A Levels), she gained three distinctions and was awarded a State Scholarship – given to the two hundred pupils who performed best in this exam in the whole country. This paid her university fees and gave her a living allowance of £80 per annum.

She gained a First in English Literature at Liverpool University, along with a prize for being the best student in her year – a leather-bound complete works of Thackeray. She also enjoyed an active social life, becoming editor of the University magazine, *The Sphinx*. At graduation, Rebecca stepped onto the platform, and the choir performed a song specially composed in her honour. 'I was there,' Naomi tells us, 'and saw and heard it.' Becky won further scholarships for postgraduate studies, becoming a research fellow at Liverpool and completing her MA on the writings of the "bluestocking" artist and author Mary Delaney. Her particular interest being eighteenth-century literature, she later amassed a collection of novels from this period.

'At home, she was always reading,' recalls Naomi, who goes on to try and trace how life started to go wrong for Becky. 'Just when she was ready to leave university, she lost the support of the people who had so far encouraged her. The Vice-Chancellor died suddenly; her professor retired to Oxford and lost interest in Liverpool. Lewis's, the department store with branches in Birmingham and Manchester, decided to start an in-house newspaper. They took [Becky] on to run it because of her experience with The Sphinx, but the experiment did not last long. She drifted for a time, then got a temporary job at Huntingdon Grammar School to replace a teacher on sick leave. She was very happy there, and appreciated her first experience of living away from home. Then mother had to go to the sanatorium; someone had to look after Fanny and all the rest of us who were still at school, so that is what she did.' In Maurice's version of events, it was her brother A.D. who, less than a year into her job, summoned her to return to Birkenhead.

Rebecca's is a curious story. It seems that, after returning home, she simply gave up on the idea of an independent career. She would have been thirty-four when her mother died, after which she did do occasional supply teaching, much of it at the newly-built Wirral Grammar School for Boys. She enjoyed this, but once the men returned from battle there were no vacancies for English teachers at the local schools. There was no evidence of any professional ambition in this extremely able woman. She relapsed into an existence of shopping, cooking and reading fiction from the local library. She lavished her affection on William, the dog Naomi had brought home as a puppy – so much so that a lot of people knew her as 'William's Missus'.

Naomi – a teacher who did succeed in mapping out a trajectory for her career – rather cruelly describes Rebecca's as 'a wasted life'. Maurice, perhaps taking their mother as his model, records that 'She had a great deal of the martyrdom complex in her… She certainly never fulfilled her academic potential and seems contented to have done all the necessary household chores, including knitting, sewing, cooking and cleaning, tasks which previously she had done only very rarely.' She bore a striking physical resemblance to Miriam, and perhaps saw herself as the replacement mother. She was the one Papperovitch indifferent to foreign travel. It is doubtful whether A.D., a keen traveller, ever invited her to accompany him on his trips. Her favourite destination was Darley Dale, where Sidney lived. She and A.D. seem to have been the only members of the family to have maintained a good relationship with his wife Margaret.

Her older sister, as Naomi recalls, 'became strange' as she aged, 'her face looked all crumpled, as though she was on the verge of tears. There was only a trace left of the happy, successful and popular young woman she had once been.' Rivkah remained physically and mentally fit until, in her early seventies, she experienced loss of vision owing to a retinal haemorrhage. This must have been a blow to such an avid reader. On 11 October 1975, excited by the prospect of a visit from Sidney's family, she went out to buy something extra for their lunch, but collapsed in the shop and died immediately (according to Naomi) or in the ambulance (if you go by Maurice's version). Rivkah's death was from heart failure (according to Maurice) or a blood clot (according to Naomi. Those two never did agree on much). Nineteen years later, Maurice, a younger brother who had once upon a time truly loved her, died on 12 October.

A.D. (Avram David)

Avram David (A.D.) was – as the eldest male – considered the most important member of the family in that generation. It was he who bought the house in Rocky Bank Road for his parents; nearly twenty years later, it was he who had the final say in the dispute over their dying father. A shy, gentle man, the experience seemed to make him retreat even further into his shell.

Born in 1904, he was, according to his father, originally named Avram Tuvia after the uncle who had drowned in Poland. 'But apparently A.D.'s elder sisters preferred the name David' – which was to become his official second name outside the family. Naomi refers to him as 'Aby', and recalls that when, at the end of his life, he went to live in a home for the elderly, he wanted to be known once more as 'David'. Whether all this name-changing suggests an identity crisis, it is hard to tell. To me, he always came across as the most phlegmatic of uncles. He had a nickname too: his brothers referred to him as 'The Stiff', because he was the tallest member of this small-framed family – and also, I suspect, because of his awkward manner. It wasn't until, in my twenties, I invited home a friend who could barely stifle his laughter when he heard Dr Pappworth referring to his brother as 'The Stiff' that it struck me as the slightest bit peculiar.

A.D., after unsatisfactory experiences at two earlier schools, gained a scholarship to the local boys' grammar school, the Birkenhead Institute, which his two younger brothers were later to attend. Like them, and also Rebecca, he moved on to the University of Liverpool, where he studied history. He went on to gain an MA in Social and Economic History, with his dissertation on the social reformer Robert Owen. Naomi recalls that when, around 1920, she entered a competition to guess the name of a doll, 'Aby' told her to suggest 'Lenin' or 'Trotsky'. 'The lady organiser was shocked and we Papperovitches were all told to go home.'

All of his siblings who took an interest in politics grew up to be proudly left-wing. A.D. lectured in social and economic history at the Workers' Education Association and the adult education branch of the University. Two or three times a week he lectured in the Blackpool area, also running classes in Liverpool and Birkenhead. By these means he succeeded in paying off his debt to Birkenhead Council, which (as he'd failed to win a state scholarship) had funded his university fees. He worked extremely hard. He does, however, seem to have found the odd moment in which to relax: there was, Naomi remembers, 'a tremendous row because something was found in Aby's pocket. Later "research" suggests that it was a packet of condoms.' But sex was a 'taboo topic' in the Papperovitch household. About menstruation the older sisters told the younger ones precisely nothing.

A.D. 'must have been a good teacher,' remarks Naomi. In an article she read in the *New Statesman* by Jack Jones, the leading trade unionist and pensioners' champion said that he owed his career to 'this brilliant teacher at the WEA who gave him his enthusiasm for working class history – named A.D. Pappworth'. All A.D.'s teaching took place in the evening; during the day he attended Liverpool University Law School. Having graduated from law school, and being exempt from army service due to a duodenal ulcer, he read for the Bar at Grays Inn under David Maxwell Fyfe, later Lord Kilmuir and Attorney General.

As a barrister, A.D. acted extensively for the trade unions, specialising in workers' compensation. An ardent Labour Party supporter throughout his life, he would never have dreamed of taking on more lucrative briefs for the employers or insurance companies. A.D. went into Chambers with Bertram B. Beras, a leading figure in Liverpool's Jewish community, and gradually built up a reasonable practice. Later he did a lot of divorce work, and was also a junior lecturer at Liverpool's Law School. He was a keen Zionist, and President of the Inter-University Student Zionist Movement. During the 1930s he was elected as a Labour Councillor in Birkenhead, taking a particular interest in libraries and art galleries, and he worked on behalf of the Labour MP for Birkenhead North, William Egan. He became friendly with the local MP Frank Soskice, later Solicitor-General in Attlee's government.

He and Rebecca/Rivkah even started to do quite a lot of entertaining at Rocky Bank Road. But when, during the 1960s, A.D. was offered the position of Alderman, he refused. A.D. played an important role in local Labour Party politics – but the only vaguely political comment I ever heard him make was disapproval of the fact that, as a student, I was living in what he called a 'slum' in east Oxford. Maurice comments: 'A.D. was never an ambitious fellow. On the contrary, he was always very self-effacing, certainly to a fault. I once asked him why he was never elected a QC, and his answer was that he had no desire to live in London, which would then become essential.' Though a reserved and modest man, he was always something of a dandy in his attire. He was the only one of the three Papperovitch sons not to marry, and was very reluctant to talk about his work. 'I suppose,' muses Naomi, 'that he never really had a chance to marry and break away to make a life for himself. The finances of the family were so dependent on his earnings.'

After Rivkah's death, he worked as a circuit judge in Lancashire, continuing to make trips to the south Yorkshire home of Sidney and Margaret, who dealt with his dirty laundry. At one point he considered going to live with them, until Maurice persuaded him to come to London. 'He was completely at a loss,' says Naomi, 'and did not know what to do with himself. He broke down and told Esther that he thought he had made a mess of his life. He should not have burdened himself with the family, taking it for granted that he should provide us all with a home.'

A.D. was of course invited to my sister Dinah's wedding in Jerusalem on 6 October 1980. But he had already arranged to go on a tour of the west coast of the US. He finally decided to go. The sisters received a postcard to say that he was enjoying the trip, though finding it 'strenuous'. He died in October 1980 at the age of seventy-six in California – found dead by a chamber-maid in his hotel bedroom in San Francisco. He was the victim, like Rivkah, of a sudden heart attack. Maurice made arrangements with the British Consul for A.D.'s body to be repatriated. He was buried in Bushey Cemetery, where London meets Hertfordshire. Naomi describes the funeral as 'horrendous. Heavy rain had fallen for days; the grave was a sea of mud. The coffin arrived from Heathrow on an old lorry. Only the immediate family and one representative of the Liverpool Bar were there.' My recollections tally with Naomi's: I vividly remember my cousin Rachel's gasp of surprise as the coffin suddenly appeared, loaded onto an ungainly cart: 'My goodness! It's The Uncle...' More than thirty years later I located his grave. A.D., I discovered, was travelling into eternity in the unassuming, almost anonymous fashion that was a mark of his personality. Weather and pollution had so eroded the stone, his name was barely visible. I said a prayer for him and left.

Esther and Leah: 'an inordinate desire to help the less fortunate'

Esther

Esther was the sibling to whom, in later life, Maurice became the closest. Born in 1906, like Hetty she left school at fourteen. She was probably the least studious of the children. In her *Chronicles*, Naomi relates that 'She was always in trouble for making unsuitable friends, for example the daughter of the milkman who lived up the road, whose main disqualification in my father's eyes was that she was not Jewish. But as he had chosen to live in a neighbourhood without Jews, she was hardly to blame for this.'

Esther initially worked for her father, to whom she often referred as 'The Gov'. Her job was to hand-sew the suit trousers, which required little skill. She spent most of her weekends at a Jewish club on the Wirral. Esther left home at the age of twenty-eight, after Rivkah accused her of hitting the bedridden Fanny and their father threw her out. This was probably an excuse for Isaac to sort out his most difficult daughter.

Esther simply wasn't like her sisters. Although lively-minded and capable, she wasn't interested in proving herself professionally, but seems to have cared more about having a good time. She was the only well-dressed Papperovitch daughter: I have a photo of her on display, wearing what looks like a ball-gown, her throat draped in pearls. She always loved jewellery. Maybe her interest in clothes and fabrics sprang from the tailoring skills she developed at her father's workshop.

Esther and her father had arguments about her habit of crossing to Liverpool every weekend to go dancing, not returning home until the early hours. Naomi recalls: 'It is extraordinary now to think of how, night after night, she caught the last ferry boat from Liverpool, at about midnight, then walked about two miles home.' There was no public transport at that time, and of course a taxi was out of the question. According to Maurice, Esther sometimes missed the last passenger boat across the Mersey, relying instead on the hourly 'luggage-boat' service, which normally carried cars only but allowed passengers to board as day broke. Naomi shared a bed with her sister, and often lay awake 'imagining what horrors might have befallen her.' Esther had a boyfriend, a slim young man called 'Tex' (Simon) Halfkin. He often came to Greenway Road. However, being the eldest child of a widowed mother, and the family's chief bread-winner, there were no marriage plans. Like Esther, Tex loved dancing.

After her final row with her father, Esther went to live with friends, near the home of Tex's mother. He was not a well man, suffering from a serious heart condition. After he had been admitted to hospital, Esther was a constant visitor. Maurice takes up the story: 'I well remember that when in 1934 [the year Esther left home] I was a resident medical officer in the Mill Road Municipal Hospital, I found [Halfkin] on my ward to my great surprise. He had extensive valvular heart disease, and died soon after that.' So Esther was the Papperovitch daughter who came closest to marrying, until tragedy intervened and she joined forever the ranks of her spinster sisters. Ironically, it was this once wayward daughter who, with Naomi, provided the home in which their father was to spend the last years of his life.

After Tex's death, Esther moved to London. In 1940 during the Blitz, when she was working for a tailor in Oxford Street, neighbours she knew well were killed in an air raid. She decided to leave London, going to stay with a friend in Manchester. But she had only just arrived when a bus hit her, leaving her with multiple injuries, including the fracture of several vertebrae. She later told Naomi that she overheard a nurse saying 'Poor girl: she won't last the night.' She had to spend six months at the Manchester Jewish Hospital and three months in convalescent homes in Southport. For a long time her whole torso was encased in plaster. Then she progressed to a padded steel frame the length of her back, until gradually she was able to walk again. For some years, the only support Esther needed was a corset – although she did later graduate to what Naomi describes as 'a fearsome surgical corset. It came from her armpits, right down her back. Only in very hot weather did she complain of the discomfort, so it was difficult to realise what she must be suffering.'

Naomi was by now working at a school in Ludlow, and in 1943 invited Esther to join her. Through a town councillor friend of Naomi's, Esther found work as a billeting officer, helping to find homes for young evacuees from East London. Naomi tells us that her sister 'loved' the job, 'and made a great success of it… forcing the local "aristocracy", in their Georgian mansions, to take in "slum" children. A testimonial from the Town Clerk records that, owing to her efforts, Ludlow held the record [in the whole country] for evacuees not returning home.' Naomi kept that testimonial, and a brief but moving account Esther wrote of her work for the Jewish Welfare Board. Esther always loved children, spending much of her later career working with them and becoming our most doting aunt.

After the war Esther applied to the London School of Economics but was unsuccessful, most places being reserved for those who had served in the Forces. Her interviewer did write on her behalf to the Charity Organisation Society, later known as the Family Welfare Association, arranging for Esther to have a six-month training course in social work in London. Although the pay was poor, Esther loved being a social worker. Esther worked very hard, becoming an expert at fundraising bazaars and jumble sales, as well as overseeing the many applications for help. When Naomi started working in London in September 1949, she and Esther set up house together in Cholmeley Park, Highgate.

It was, according to Naomi's account, 'with reluctance' that Esther applied for a job on the staff of the Jewish Board of Guardians, which became the Jewish Welfare Board and then Jewish Care. 'But the pay was about double the pittance she got at FWA; there was also a pension.' Most of her career with the Board involved working with the elderly at homes in London, Southend, Brighton and Bournemouth, where there were Jewish communities, including many retired people. When she reached the Board's compulsory retirement age, this energetic woman joined the Eleanor Rathbone Society, looking after mothers and children who, in those days, were called 'educationally sub-normal'; now 'special needs.' She helped them to make clothes for themselves and their children, and took them on outings. When this job finished, she did voluntary work at a Jewish old people's home and kept busy with a local club for pensioners. She continued well into old age to volunteer at the League of Jewish Women and the International Council of Women. During my gap year she arranged for me to do voluntary work one-to-one with an 'ESN' child, Brian, and also basic nursery nursing at a Jewish home for babies and young children.

Esther couldn't sit still, and was possibly the only Papperovitch unlikely to be found with a book in her hand. Maurice comments: 'This history is proof, if such were needed, that Esther is a person of great compassion and with an inordinate desire to help the less fortunate.' She certainly tried to help him as much as she could when his marriage was foundering. She suffered in her later years from rheumatism, and also developed a heart condition, being looked after at the Royal Free Hospital by my father's consultant. She died in April 1992, aged eighty-six, a month after our son Adam was born. Naomi was at her hospital bedside when she died.

Leah

Of all the Papperovitch siblings, Leah – born in 1908 – was the most successful in detaching herself from the family and creating her own life independent of its eccentricities. Leaving school (like Hetty and Esther) aged fourteen, she wanted to study art in Liverpool, but there were no scholarships for this, and no money available to pay the fees. 'In any case,' recalls Naomi, 'my parents and the siblings thought it was a daft idea.' So she had to make do with evening classes in art. For a time she was apprenticed to a dressmaker. Then, like Esther, she went on to work for her father, doing the hand-sewing on the trousers: stitching the lining of the waistband, putting on the buttons and making button holes. When her father had no work (which was often the case), Leah went to people's houses to make their curtains and repair their linen. She also had an arrangement with a local private school to make their shoe bags.

All Leah's spare time was spent at Beechcroft, an adult education settlement. She attended several different kinds of craft classes and tried to learn German. But her main interest was in amateur dramatics. She was given some small parts, and frequently employed as a prompter and (naturally) a costume maker. Sundays saw her out with the Ramblers' Association, walking in North Wales and Derbyshire, and she also went on climbing holidays. 'For some reason,' Naomi recalls, 'these activities were made fun of by the rest of the family. She accepted her position as the fool of the family.'

She remained close to Esther and Naomi, the latter especially. But whereas other members of the family travelled on a north-south trajectory along England, she ventured east and west, living first near Worcester, then in Norwich, and finally settling in Bristol. She always chose interesting cities with a lively cultural scene, and set in attractive countryside.

On the outbreak of war, Leah chose to join the Land Army. She was sent to the forestry division in Shropshire, a few miles from Ludlow where Esther and Naomi worked during the war. Leah loved village life and the beautiful countryside around her. Naomi used to cycle up to visit her most weekends, or Leah came down to Ludlow. When the Land Army was disbanded, Leah did not want to return to Birkenhead. Fortunately, she was accepted onto a new government training scheme to make up for the shortage of teachers, and worked initially at Worcester Technical College where she taught dressmaking and soft furnishing.

She then found a job in Norwich, where she soon had a circle of friends, including members of the synagogue. She lived in a comfortable flat in a modern block. 'She was very happy there,' according to Naomi. But when the local authority decided to change the institution into a technical college, Leah's working life changed. She was transferred to a tough comprehensive school. This quietly-spoken young woman found she could not cope with the discipline. So she got a job at a girls' school in Bristol, where she worked until her retirement. Her speciality was needlework – the subject she taught at school. But in Bristol she also conducted evening classes in leatherwork, dressmaking and pattern-making. For several years she volunteered in the wardrobe department at the Bristol Old Vic. A founding and active member of Bristol's Progressive Synagogue, she made many friends in the area.

Like so many of her siblings, Leah was a natural teacher: I recall her patiently helping our nieces with some children's needlework they had brought along to a family celebration. And, in her retirement, Leah was as Naomi puts it, 'able to fulfil the ambition of her youth: she learned to paint.' I still have on the wall two oil paintings she gave me: a still life and a Cornish village. She and Naomi enjoyed going on holiday together both in this country and abroad.

She had reached a modest level of prosperity that might have surprised the brothers and sisters who used to tease her. 'It was very much to her credit,' remarks Naomi, 'that she was able to put together enough money to buy a pleasant flat in Clifton and to furnish it comfortably'.

For several of the Pappworth siblings, brought up in such a sparse and unappealing house, matters of home and furniture remained permanently important. Leah was, according to her younger sister, 'immensely house-proud, which made clearing up after her death especially painful. Among the accumulation of a lifetime... I found a bundle of love letters. I read only the beginning of the top one, enough to realise what they were. Then I destroyed them. This was a side of her life which she never confided to me. I thought it best that it should remain her secret.'

Leah's old age (she lived into her mid-eighties) was very hard. She was plagued with persistent backache owing to osteoporosis. She claimed to Maurice that this condition had caused her to lose nine inches in height. I was very struck by the way, each time I saw her, she seemed to have shrunk: she became a very tiny woman with a hunched back. At the end, as Naomi put it, 'she turned her face to the wall'. Whatever the clinical cause of death, she had resolved it was time to go. Always a determined woman, she carried out this final decision without fuss.

Sidney and Naomi: achievement and rivalry

Sidney

Maurice's relationship with the sibling closest in age to him was complicated. During the second half of his life, his feelings towards Sidney were very ambivalent. But as children, with Sidney (born in June 1911) only seventeen months Maurice's junior, the two boys were inseparable. They were often taken for twins, Sidney being the taller. According to Naomi, Maurice compensated for his small size by being 'something of a bully'.

In his memoir, Maurice rather brutally remarks of his brother's school career: 'he won a half scholarship to the local boys' grammar school. This meant that he had not sufficiently impressed those who had interviewed him for admission... to be awarded a full scholarship' – unlike Maurice himself, of course. The importance of scholarships rode high, there being little spare money for the luxury of school fees. But Isaac's provision of half of Sidney's fees was certainly a good investment: the latter did well at Matriculation and Higher School Certificate, gaining a place at Liverpool Medical School, in the year below Maurice, and qualifying in June 1933. Maurice characteristically offers the information that his younger brother 'did not do particularly well...in the professional examinations.' He chose not to mention the fact that Sidney came second out of all those taking the Royal College of Surgeons examination. According to Sidney's family, Maurice's response was that he should have been placed first, only the prevalent anti-Semitism standing in his way.

But, as Naomi remarks, 'Maurice was a "swot," while Sidney appeared to take his studies lightly, doing quite well with apparently little effort.' While studying at Liverpool, both boys continued to live at home. 'Every evening,' Naomi tells us, 'Maurice sat at the kitchen table with his books, demanding silence from the rest of the family. Getting a houseman's job was their first experience of living away from home.' Even then, they were still in Liverpool.

Sidney's first appointment was as a casualty officer at the Liverpool Royal Infirmary; after the war, he became a demonstrator in Anatomy at Liverpool University, where he trained as an orthopaedic surgeon. Maurice has the grace to describe this department at Liverpool as 'the pioneer and most famous school of orthopaedics certainly in the UK, if not in the entire world'. The school was run by Sir Robert Jones, whose work greatly impressed Sidney and helped him to decide that this would be his specialist area. Having gained a Mastership of Surgery in Orthopaedics, Sidney became a registrar at Sheffield Royal Infirmary.

Sidney was the most free-and-easy of the Papperovitch children. The first car he bought was a second-hand MG sports, rather different from what Maurice considered his own 'sedate second-hand car purchases'. I have a photo of the three Papperovitch brothers gazing at it in admiration.

During that first job in casualty at Liverpool Royal Infirmary, he decided to spend his allocated holiday on a cruise to Norway. But the fjords had to wait: soon after boarding, Sidney injured his leg in the dark, and was returned to shore, to be admitted to his workplace with a severe leg infection. It took a long time to heal. Maurice, one feels, may have believed that his younger brother had got his comeuppance for being simply too adventurous. He did intervene and arrange for the Professor of Clinical Medicine to examine his brother. The subsequent diagnosis was ulcerative colitis – one of those recurring Papperovitch diseases.

On the outbreak of war, having made a satisfactory recovery, Sidney volunteered for service in the Royal Army Medical Corps. 'Even more surprisingly,' remarks his brother, 'he was accepted.' He served in Hertfordshire and Ireland, but had to be discharged soon after Dunkirk, when his ulcerative colitis recurred. But Sidney had his moments of good fortune, notably his survival of an air raid, when a bomb fell on his operating theatre, killing several colleagues.

Another piece of luck for Sidney occurred while he was working as an orthopaedic registrar in Sheffield. Here he met a house surgeon called Margaret Curtis. Sidney married her in a register office without telling anyone in the family. Margaret later converted to Judaism, having undergone a course of instruction and learned to read Hebrew. There then followed the 'official' wedding at the Sheffield Orthodox Synagogue, which Isaac attended. He enjoyed spending weekends at Sidney and Margaret's home in Darley Dale, Derbyshire, especially after the birth of their first child (and his eldest grandchild), Peninnah. Theirs was a large stone house with several acres of grounds, from which they later moved to another rural house about ten miles from Sheffield.

Sidney was by now a consultant orthopaedic surgeon at the Northern Sheffield Hospital. He and Margaret kept dogs and horses, settling into a lifestyle far removed from that of Sidney's upbringing. Peninnah and Rachel were sent as boarders to that most English of establishments, Cheltenham Ladies' College, which they both disliked. Their younger brother Adam boarded at Westminster. Peninnah married a non-Jewish boy she met while studying at the University of Leeds. So her parents' pattern was repeated. But Stephen was not the kind of young man to convert, and there was for some years an estrangement between Sidney and Margaret and their elder daughter. By the time they all attended our wedding in 1982, they had been reconciled. Peninnah has six children, the youngest, Aaron, with her partner Colm McAllister (she and Stephen divorced while her first four were still very young). Having lived in Bristol for many years, Peninnah moved back north, settling near Darlington. Trained as an accountant, she switched to education and became a head teacher. So the pedagogic family trend continued.

Rachel ventured further afield. Having made an unsuccessful start to studying medicine, she branched out into engineering – an unusual path for young women in the 1970s – and moved to Houston, Texas. There she became a successful oil consultant, advising firms on ecologically friendly production methods. She married a Christian Iraqi widower, Mudafeh el Saleh, whose previous wife had also been Jewish. With him she has two children. Adam became a solicitor, and has done much of his legal work in Gibraltar. Despite Maurice and Sidney's estrangement, their five daughters are in regular touch, attending family celebrations and memorials, and laying past conflicts to rest.

It wasn't just their disagreement over how to treat their gravely ill father that caused the rift between Maurice and Sidney. The problems continued when the two brothers got married: their wives didn't get on. Jean apparently found Margaret intimidating because she would demonstrate her skills in cookery, knitting, crocheting – all areas in which Jean had not the slightest interest. Esther, the sister to whom Maurice was closest at this time, felt a strong antipathy towards Margaret, which she was never able to explain. The feeling was mutual. Margaret was to become a national advisor on family planning. Later, she developed acute peripheral neuritis and then glaucoma, and sought Maurice's advice as she was dissatisfied with her care. So you could say there was some sort of reconciliation between the two brothers towards the end. But it is a sad story of companionship turned to rivalry and life choices that, despite their shared profession, sent them on strongly divergent paths.

Naomi

The youngest in the family, Naomi was the sibling with whom Maurice had the most mutually antipathetic relationship. Both were strong, clever and obstinate characters, destined to clash. Naomi was born in December 1915. Like Maurice, she was very influenced by their older sister Rebecca-Rivkah, who virtually brought them up. Rivkah's revelation to Naomi of the delights of English literature was evidently passed on to the other three youngest members of the family. In her *Chapters of Autobiography*, Naomi reminisces: 'We played guessing games, shouting the answers from room to room. A favourite one was guessing the author of first lines of poetry. Palgrave's *Golden Treasury* was the main source, and my memory is still stuffed with first lines although I have forgotten the rest of the poems.' I find it very moving to picture these four children, the youngest in an aspirational immigrant family, penetrating the culture of their parents' adopted country through these kind of games. John Donne became one of Naomi's favourite poets, to whom she introduced me when I was preparing for my Oxford entrance exams. Indeed, if it weren't for Naomi I would never have gone to Oxford. I remember standing with her in 1972 in her bedroom in her Highgate flat, looking through her window all the way up to

Alexandra Palace, as she suggested I should give Oxford a try. My school never encouraged me. I followed in her footsteps and went to St Hugh's.

Naomi was a very bright child, perhaps partly as a result of having observed and absorbed so much from her eight elder siblings. She came top in the entrance exam to Birkenhead High School, where she was awarded a scholarship. At this time, the summer of 1927, she felt very happy. One evening, she recalls in her *Chapters of Autobiography*, 'Esther exclaimed in astonishment, "Whatever happened to you? You look as though you are going to explode." And that was how I felt. I had a light inside me.' Naomi's experience of Birkenhead High was not, however, particularly happy, partly because of her sense that, poor and Jewish, she was so very different from the other girls. She did beg her mother for the money to buy all the vital High School girl's kit, such as lacrosse stick and boots, tennis racquet, textbooks. Her mother in turn 'begged my eldest brother... Hetty provided money for spectacles.'

One especially revealing passage in Naomi's memoir describes what one might call her ideal family. This was the family of her Birkenhead High School friend, Lavinia, who shared Naomi's humble background: 'Her father was a manual labourer, and her parents and three sisters lived in a tiny terraced house in a slum area of the town, but it was the happiest family I have ever met. The parents had married young, and they demonstrably loved each other and their four daughters... The house was full of laughter and affection.'

Naomi gained three distinctions at Higher School Certificate, and in 1934 was awarded a state scholarship and an additional college scholarship to Oxford to read Modern History. She initially applied to Somerville, who didn't award her a scholarship. St Hugh's did, and her time there was certainly much happier than her years at school. Maurice was actively helpful in her Oxford application, as Naomi acknowledges: 'A credit in maths was then essential for matriculation, and without his help [the maths teaching at Birkenhead High being poor], I could not have achieved this – not that I ever understood what quadratic equations were for.'

After gaining her history degree at Oxford, Naomi drifted into teaching, more with a sense of it being her best possible option than from a deep vocational urge. Her first post was at High Wycombe Girls' Grammar School. To her surprise, Naomi found that she enjoyed teaching, and was good at it. During the war she taught at the Girls' Grammar School in Ludlow, which she loved, but then moved to London, where she worked at the Cooper School in the Mile End Road. She was Head of History at Brondesbury and Kilburn High School for Girls, a direct grant school, which in the 1960s amalgamated with Kilburn High School for Boys to become a comprehensive. A Labour Party member all her life until Tony Blair authorised the invasion of Iraq in 2003 (aged nearly ninety, she was visited by her local Labour MP when she resigned her Party membership), Naomi swallowed hard and put up with the deterioration of her once high-achieving school.

Unlike her siblings, she loved talking about her work, and regaled her nieces with stories about the various characters and minor disasters that coloured her life at school. She was a tiny woman, who, on seeing a 'Back to School' sign in a local shop, marched in and bought herself a pair of children's shoes: she was a size 2. But she was also formidable, and I wouldn't have wanted to be a pupil who had displeased her. She was clearly a brilliant teacher (who helped me write rather a good O Level essay on the French Revolution) – and also a pioneering one. At a time when very few schools offered cultural trips abroad, she took groups of girls to Florence in 1968, Rome in 1970 and Madrid in 1971, organising the itinerary herself and giving highly knowledgeable tours of churches, palaces and galleries. Dinah and I joined the trip to Florence, and I was also on the visit to Madrid. Esther always accompanied, her chief role being to do battle with the young Italian and Spanish men who pursued such an enticing troop of girls.

Maurice's account of Naomi in his taped autobiography is much briefer than that of any of his other siblings. 'I personally have always found her an extremely selfish person, concerned entirely with her own self and so completely unlike Esther'. Esther was probably *too* unselfish; Naomi was selfish chiefly in that she was determined to create her own life and not to follow the example of Rivkah, her most intellectually gifted sister, in giving it all up to look after someone else. Perhaps this is why she never married; certainly she found physical contact difficult, and even verbally seemed unable to express affection. But she became very fond of Peninnah and her children, and, after Esther's death, grew close to my sister Sara's children, who lived nearby.

Having been healthy and active, Naomi was in her seventies struck by the heart disease that had killed A.D. and Rivkah, and had already been diagnosed in Maurice. About to board a train to visit a friend in Shropshire, she suffered a heart attack at Euston station, from where she was taken to University College Hospital. Naomi made a good recovery, and stayed on medication for the rest of her life. After Esther's death in 1992, she lived on for nearly fourteen years at the Cholmeley Lodge flat in Highgate. She was undoubtedly lonely, and her quite severe deafness must have left her feeling particularly isolated. Towards the end of her life, she had the unsettling experience of finding in herself exactly the symptoms from which her father suffered in his final year.

Her circulation was failing, the blood supply having problems in reaching her feet and lower legs. Always tiny, she had the weight of a child. She felt the cold badly: I remember giving her thermal vests for her ninetieth birthday. Her lower limbs were in danger of gangrene. The Whittington Hospital was able to offer Naomi an operation which, she was told, couldn't be guaranteed to work and did contain risks – particularly for a ninety-year-old. She was worried and frightened but decided to go ahead with the operation; there were complications; she died in hospital.

Naomi loved Waterlow Park, just a few minutes' walk from her Highgate home. For years she would walk through this park on her way to Gospel Oak station, from where she would catch the train to her day's teaching in Kilburn. Sara and I found a beautiful spot for a bench commemorating her life. It bears a quotation from Andrew Marvell's 'The Garden'. Naomi it was who introduced me, nearly thirty-four years earlier, to the Metaphysical Poets. This was the legacy of one who, like the brother who couldn't trust her, was a truly great teacher.

'It is so difficult to die': parents leave, brothers clash

Maurice's mother Miriam died in February 1935 at the age of sixty-three. According to Maurice, it was in 1929, six months after the death from tuberculosis at the age of only thirty of her second daughter Fanny, that Miriam developed a chest infection. Naomi, however, insists that their mother started coughing before 1927. In the *Chronicles*, Naomi records how 'I used to lie in bed in the attic and listen to her and pray, "Please God, don't let Mother have consumption"… I was frightened.'

When the doctor was eventually called, he confirmed that this coughing was indeed a symptom of 'consumption,' or tuberculosis. Maurice, stepping forward with his diagnosis, states 'there can be no doubt that she had contracted it from Fanny, whom she had lovingly nursed during her last months of illness'. Miriam was sent to a sanatorium in Delamere, in a rural part of Cheshire. Here her health showed signs of improvement, but – unable to read the letters in English sent to her from home – she felt isolated and unhappy. Once she was

back home, Miriam's health continued to be unreliable: she had frequent re-
lapses, especially in winter. Though she no longer coughed up blood, the disease remained in her lungs. The worst of these occurred in 1934, when continuing fever forced this temperamentally energetic woman to remain in bed. She
had been trying to continue with the household chores, with some help from a
young girl who came in to clean, paid for by A.D., who was by now earning
some money as lecturer.

Not one of the daughters was at home to look after their mother, until Rebecca (daughter number three) left her English teaching job in Huntingdon at
A.D.'s urgent request, and came to live in Rocky Bank Road. Rebecca/Rivkah
never returned to her job, remaining in Rocky Bank Road for the rest of her life.
Not long after she gave up her post, the mother she had come back to nurse
died: on 2 February 1935, aged sixty-three. Miriam's husband went on to reach
the age of eighty-eight.

Naomi was a student at Oxford when her mother died. On the train back,
she recalls, 'I read steadily [Virginia Woolf's] *The Waves*... I did not take in a
word that I read. I have never subsequently opened the book.' Walking towards
the family home in Rocky Bank Road, 'I told myself that if there was a light in
the bay window of her room, it would not be true that Mother was dead. There
was a light, but I knew that it was true... The funeral was in Liverpool, in a
horrid, mean cemetery near a railway line. As we waited for the hearse, my
father cried.'

So the *ayshet chayil* gave her life for one of her children – a life of tough
physical labour, with who knows what thoughts inside her head. I have a photograph of her leaning against a mantelpiece by a vase of flowers (I still have
the vase). Her lips – whose shape my father and I inherited – are tight shut but
smiling, and her eyes, sparkling from creased folds, are smiling too. She seems
to be enjoying a private joke with herself.

According to Maurice's memoir, his mother's death was 'a terrible blow'
to Isaac: 'for a long time he was depressed and appeared to have very little
interest in life. He did not get up till midday and after making himself breakfast
he went off for walks to the local parks or to Liverpool.' So his decision to
move away from Birkenhead, which coincided with Hetty's fatal illness, came
as little surprise.

During the early 1950s, Isaac travelled to London to stay with Esther and
Naomi, sharing their flat in Highgate so that he could more easily visit his eldest
child, Hetty, in Bournemouth. After several visits to London, he decided he

wasn't going to return to Birkenhead. Isaac did indeed move south for the remaining eight years or so of his life. He stayed with Esther and Naomi in Highgate so that he could travel down to Hetty; Maurice came to visit. Then Isaac had his first heart attack. Maurice paid for a nurse to come in daily during the week, and the two sisters took over when they returned from work in the evening. Their father recovered, but never returned to Birkenhead. 'Rivkah,' Naomi writes, 'made it clear that she did not want him back.'

When Esther, Naomi and Isaac moved to another Highgate flat just up the road in Cholmeley Lodge, he shared a bedroom with Esther. According to Maurice, he settled well into his new life, becoming very involved in the Highgate Synagogue on Archway Road. This involved a steep walk back up the hill, which eventually became too much for him. Naomi confesses that her 'final distaste for orthodox Judaism came when the local rabbi told us that he would rather Dad didn't go to synagogue at all, than in a car on Shabbas'. My own father, similarly afflicted by a heart condition in later life, was given exactly the same advice by his rabbi. Of Isaac's six grandchildren, only one remains in the orthodox fold.

Isaac loved spending time in nearby Waterlow Park, and later even walked across the Heath to Hampstead to visit us at our home in Keats Grove. He had much enjoyed Maurice's wedding to Jean, with whom he got on very well. She recalled that he was at first rather confused when she bent over to kiss his cheek, but grew to enjoy this unaccustomed experience. He also visited his only other married child, Sidney, in Darley Dale.

He also spent time reading – in Yiddish, naturally. Maurice recalls him reading the whole of *War and Peace* in this way. He enjoyed historical novels, which Esther brought home for him from the Whitechapel Public Library, which still retained a section of books in Yiddish. The Yiddish stories her father read in this way were printed in Hebrew characters, which his religious education had ensured he was able to read. Maurice bought him a television set. His favourite programmes were *Emergency Ward 10* (which I remember watching with him) and the serialisation of Dorothy L. Sayers' *The Man Born to be King*. 'He did not realise,' explains Naomi, 'that the hero was the Jesus Christ we had always been forbidden to name.'

Britain swung into the Sixties when Isaac developed angina, and also calf pain on walking. His symptoms were at first considered to be simply part of the ageing process. As it turned out, they were to run through his children as part of the family heritage. 'At the beginning of September 1960,' records Maurice, 'while in my Harley Street consulting room, I had a message from Naomi that Dad was complaining of very severe pain in both legs.' Maurice went up to Highgate to examine his father. He realised immediately that his condition was serious. Keeping strictly to the medical etiquette of not treating family members, he asked Naomi to telephone Dr Alec Philips, an East End GP and a close friend of Esther's. Alec ordered an ambulance and had Isaac admitted to the Whittington Hospital. He had a blockage due to a blood clot at the distal end of the main abdominal artery where it divides into the right and left main arteries supplying both lower limbs.

Maurice telephoned A.D. and Rivkah, who came to London that evening, along with Sidney and his wife Margaret. He records that 'In 1960 vascular surgery was in its infancy, and it was considered… that Dad would not survive any attempt to remove that blood clot. But by next morning there was gross circulatory deficiency in both lower limbs. The consultant expressed his opinion that because the legs were gangrenous [any attempt to remove the clot] would be fatal, and the only chance was for him to have amputations of both lower limbs. By this time Dad was only semi-conscious and unable to give his opinion, let alone consent. I was opposed to such surgery. I could not contemplate Dad recovering consciousness after such surgery and finding he had no lower limbs.'

However Sidney, as an orthopaedic surgeon, strongly supported the operation. 'The consultant decided that the final decision should be given by A.D., who supported my view. Father was given adequate morphine to control the pain and, as I wished, we let him die in peace. This incident and the controversy had a major lasting effect on me personally. I discussed this several times with distinguished physicians, who all agreed with my decision. Father died on 11 September 1960, aged eighty-eight.'

At a personal level, not only did Maurice lose his father, but also – in effect – the brother who, only seventeen months younger than himself, had been his closest childhood companion. It is obviously difficult if siblings are both doctors and disagree on what is best for their gravely ill parent. Naomi remembers Isaac saying, 'It is so difficult to die', and 'My life has passed like a dream.'

Sidney's daughters Peninnah and Rachel stopped off in London with their parents and brother Adam to visit their grandfather in hospital. Peninnah has a vivid recollection of the breach between her father and mine: 'I can remember going to see my grandfather, who was in a single room in the hospital, and my mother talking kindly to him, patting his hand and telling him that he would be

OK and that she and Sidney would look after him; he was not to worry. The next thing I recall is that I was coming down a staircase... and my mother was having a loud argument with Maurice who was higher up on the stairs... what I understood is that my parents wanted my grandfather to have an operation but that other relatives didn't agree and that my mother charged these relatives with leaving grandfather to die a terrible death.'

Margaret, Sidney's wife, talked to Peninnah many years later about this memory. As a former orthopaedic surgeon herself, who throughout her life championed the rights of the disabled, Margaret still felt that her father-in-law would have had a good chance of survival after amputation. She offered him a home in Yorkshire with her and Sidney. But she encountered rigid hostility. Apparently Margaret, whom her daughter describes as 'really formidable when she felt strongly about something,' intervened after A.D. had announced his decision, trying to make him change his mind. She and Sidney considered 'the Uncle' (as their children called him) to have been weak. As they saw it, he had succumbed to Maurice's arguments. Maurice could certainly be as persistently persuasive as his sister-in-law. Arguably, A.D. showed great strength in standing his ground under pressure.

Whatever the merits of the two opposing opinions, this disagreement on such a serious subject severed the two brothers almost to the end of Maurice's life. Peninnah believes that 'my father eventually called my mother away, saying "Leave it, Margaret..."' She continues: 'I think the whole point of my parents' standpoint was that it [was] for the patient to make an informed choice.'

Ironically, this last sentence foreshadows the ideas at the heart of Maurice Pappworth's writing on medical ethics. Indeed, the experience of his father's final illness shows us so much about the man who, seven years later, was to publish *Human Guinea Pigs*. As the book makes clear, Maurice Pappworth put the patient and his quality of life above all else. He was wary of risky intervention and troubled by over-enthusiastic doctors. My grandfather, a semi-conscious eighty-eight-year-old, was at that moment a perfect example of the vulnerable patient whose dignity and best interests his middle son was to champion in *Human Guinea Pigs*.

Chapter Three

Prejudice and pride: a doctor at war and peace

'Wadsworth hailed me with a barrage of criticisms of Professor Cohen, and made a dismissive statement that he considered, to use his actual words, "No Jew can ever be a gentleman and I do not want one working with me."'

(from Maurice Pappworth's memoir)

Collisions with the system

Maurice Pappworth's account of his early medical posts shows someone who, from the start, encountered difficulties. Once he was qualified in 1932, he applied for one of three vacant house physician posts at the Liverpool Royal Infirmary. He was offered none of them. The reason he gives for this lack of success is that it was 'entirely due to favouritism in the case of two of the applicants. One lived in Blundellsands, a smart suburb just outside Liverpool, and knew the family of the consultant physicians who also lived there; the other played rugby for the University and had been President of the Medical Students' Society.' There may well have been other reasons why Pappworth was not offered this job, for which he was obviously very well qualified. But he was never socially polished, and was often unable to see that comments intended to be witty could be interpreted as poor taste. He may simply have been too outspoken at interview. If the medical establishment during and well beyond the 1930s was a 'club', it was one Pappworth was always going to have difficulty in joining.

Instead, Pappworth was offered the post of Combined Casualty Officer and House Surgeon to the Ear, Nose and Throat department at the Liverpool Royal Infirmary. 'I enjoyed the latter part of the job,' he concedes, 'because it enabled me to become proficient in using the necessary instruments for examining ears, noses and throats, including the vocal cords. This stood me in very good stead in later years.' He carefully records his salary – £60 per annum plus board and lodging. He also notes that at some of the London teaching hospitals, resident junior doctors were not paid at all. His interpretation of this exploitation was

54

that the privilege of working at teaching hospitals was, throughout the United Kingdom, deemed an 'adequate reward.'

After six months in Casualty and the ENT departments, he failed to get a job as a house physician at the Royal Infirmary, where he had completed almost all his 'clinical stewardship'. Just as he was deciding that it was a waste of time applying for other Liverpool jobs, he was appointed Resident Medical Officer at the Bootle General Hospital, also known as the Mill Road Infirmary, and one of the Liverpool's three municipal hospitals. Here Pappworth earned £100 a year with board and lodging, and spent 'a very enjoyable and extremely valuable' twelve months.

One of Pappworth's most influential mentors at Liverpool's School of Medicine had been Henry Cohen, who was to become Chair of Medicine in 1934. They had both attended Birkenhead Institute, and the two families were acquainted. Then, in January 1935, Pappworth was appointed to what looked like the perfect job, which promised to be an important step in his medical career. For nearly four years he was Cohen's Medical Tutor and Registrar. Pappworth assisted at Cohen's outpatient clinics at the Liverpool Royal Infirmary, conducting them himself when Cohen was away. Another senior colleague for whom he subbed in cases of absence was the dermatologist Dr Stopford Taylor. Pappworth was determined that his medical experience should be as broad as possible. As he was very friendly with some of the hospital's radiologists, he was allowed unofficially to attend their tutorials for the Diploma in Radiology. As Liverpool was one of the first hospitals in the UK to use X-rays medically, and a pioneer in this diploma course, it was clearly a good opportunity. For his paid work with Cohen, Pappworth's salary was £200 a year. To top up this salary, and in addition to his routine teaching in the wards and the outpatient department, he offered private coaching. This he gave to some of the final year students preparing for their M.B, as well as to postgraduates working for their MRCP or MD examinations. He also had a paid post in the Pharmacology Department, most of which – rather ironically – consisted of assistance with its work testing drugs on animals. It also included private tuition in pharmacology over three years for groups of ten to twelve students.

Pappworth remained with Henry Cohen as Registrar and Tutor until October 1938. The two later became estranged, as Cohen felt he couldn't condone what he considered muck-raking in *Human Guinea Pigs*. Looking back at his hugely varied experiences at the Liverpool Royal Infirmary, Pappworth comments that they 'produced an extensive breadth to my medical knowledge and abilities'. They contributed to his flowering as one of the great general physicians of his day and also, he claimed, 'helped me enormously with my Membership coaching.' He goes on to observe, in the memoir recorded during the late 1980s, that 'Nowadays this would be frowned upon, because narrow specialisation very soon after qualification is the rule.'

By 1939, Pappworth was ready for a move. A vacancy had occurred at the Stanley, the smallest of Liverpool's four teaching hospitals. What Pappworth encountered during his application for this post was to have a significant effect on how he came to view the British medical establishment, and the strategies he adopted for his career. The job title was Honorary Assistant Physician. It involved working with the Stanley's one Senior Consultant Physician, Dr Wadsworth.

Pappworth took enormous trouble with his application, which was printed in a bound booklet. After drawing attention to his successful teaching and clinical experience, he adds: 'If I am successful in this application my sincerest aim at all times will be to co-operate with the Staff in upholding the great traditions of the Liverpool Voluntary Hospitals and the welfare of their patients.' Finally, before listing two co-authored publications in medical journals, and those on which he was currently working, he refers again to teaching students as 'one of my main interests'. He points out that the number of candidates he had privately coached nearly reached one hundred, 'with a hundred per cent success. Of the fifty-eight students who sat the final M.B. examination at Liverpool last July, I had privately coached no fewer than twenty-three.' Pappworth gave the names of three referees, none of them Professor Henry Cohen.

Pappworth gives a detailed account of his interview with potential boss, Dr Wadsworth, and also refers to a discussion he had afterwards with Henry Cohen. Dr Wadsworth 'was of fairly short stature, almost as wide as he was tall, and his hair was always very closely cropped. He looked like a Prussian officer.' To Pappworth's amazement, 'Wadsworth hailed me with a barrage of criticisms of Professor Cohen, and made a dismissive statement that he considered, to use his actual words, "No Jew can ever be a gentleman and I do not want one working with me." The main reason for Wadsworth's virulence was because, when a consultant assistant physician post became vacant at the prestigious Liverpool Royal Infirmary, Cohen – who was much his junior – was appointed instead of him.'

During his later talk with Henry Cohen, 'his comment was that Wadsworth was an unsuccessful, unpleasant man, and I should not want to work with him as his assistant at any time… He was further of the opinion that I confused anti-Semitism with anti-Cohenism, to which I could not give the obvious appropriate comment – that anti-Cohenism, which was rife in the medical profession in Liverpool mainly due to envy and jealousy at his success, itself caused anti-Semitism.' At the appointments committee, which Cohen declined to attend, Pappworth had the support of Sir Robert Kelly, 'who was then Professor of Clinical Surgery and Vice-President of the Royal College of Surgeons, and a great gentleman. He was shocked by my story'. The only other applicants were a Dr Sutton and Dr John Hay Jr, 'both of whom I myself had recently successfully coached privately for the MRCP. Although Sutton was four years my junior and had only a mediocre postgraduate appointment, he was successful. Later, when a consultant vacancy did occur at the Liverpool Royal Infirmary, he was appointed to that.'

It is not just the stark testament to anti-Semitism that makes this record so disturbing. It is also the way in which, fifty years later, Pappworth was so clearly still tortured by the prejudice; the entanglement of anti-Semitism and anti-Cohenism; the memory of who helped him and who didn't; his conviction that issues other than competence governed medical appointments; even his likening of the anti-Semite to a Prussian officer. The whole experience continued to run deep and dark. Everywhere he looked, according to his brother Sidney, he found anti-Semitism.

In her 2011 interview with Professor Allan Gaw, Helen Bamber mused that many Jews in professional settings 'were not admired very much, and were not encouraged and were very often not chosen'. Bamber claimed in her interview that anti-Semitism in the 1950s and 1960s remained 'very persistent… I was involved in another position at another hospital that [shall] remain nameless, and I listened to the doctors talking about the applicants for a job, and they clearly were not going to, if they could avoid it, have another Jew… That was an enormous prejudice.'

Bamber was in no doubt that Pappworth would have experienced anti-Semitism in Liverpool. That there was inherent racism in the medical profession during Pappworth's career is considered by some to be irrefutable. Immigrant Jewish doctors from the East End, for example, found that their wartime experience fighting in the Polish army made as little impression on their medical superiors as it would make on Pappworth's. They were simply told they would never get a hospital job and should content themselves with working as GPs. One young Polish doctor working in the UK was told by a consultant that he would not land a job unless he changed his name from Kadinski. So he re-invented himself and became Sir Stanford Cade, a leading orthopaedic surgeon for young people with cancer. This dismissive attitude was meted out also to Indian doctors in the UK at this time. Jobs and promotions were just harder to come by if you didn't fit the mould.

It wasn't until several years after the publication in 1967 of *Human Guinea Pigs* that St Bartholomew's Hospital appointed its first ever Jewish surgeon. Jewish medical students tended to play safe, studying primarily at University College Hospital and the Middlesex. During the post-war years, where a doctor had trained took on disproportionate and snobbish significance: were you a Guy's man or a Thomas's man? The understanding was that doctors would re-turn later to a post at their *alma mater*. Senior consultants would groom a par-ticular junior colleague to take over their job. So, years before they came up, many jobs were simply closed off. This world of patronage was not the world of Maurice Pappworth.

But neither anti-Semitism nor nepotism explains the whole story. In Pap-pworth's case, his awkward personality was as much of a hindrance as his race and his background. And combative people who speak their mind are not gen-erally those who are most conventionally successful. Interestingly, one Jewish medical professor I interviewed had not realised that Pappworth was Jewish. Pappworth was fair-haired, and not what the general bias would consider 'Jew-ish' in his appearance. He certainly made no secret of his Judaism in his writing – but that came later in his career. For the small young man lacking in the social graces of his southern, often publicly-educated rivals for jobs, life was always going to be a challenge – in the medical profession and beyond. He must have learned something from this sense that there were so few people there to support him, determining to be more generous and helpful than many he had encoun-tered. One former MRCP student described him as a very kind man, who as-sisted her when she was looking for a job. Once he had become established, he went out of his way to guide young doctors up the greasy pole – although a name as controversial as Pappworth's later became was not necessarily the one to use when grovelling to the establishment.

After a long association with the Liverpool Royal Infirmary as undergrad-uate, resident Tutor and Registrar, Pappworth decided to pull up his northern roots and apply for posts in the south of England. It had never been part of his long-term plan that he should remain on Merseyside for the rest of his career; he was an unattached bachelor, and responded readily to the lure of London.

The pinnacle in British medicine was to become a consultant in a London teaching hospital. There was without doubt plenty of nepotism, and very little regulation of the appointments system. And there existed, as one eminent professor phrased it in conversation, a 'lineage' of doctors. Even the application for medical school was unfair: candidates had to state what their parents' jobs were. Newly-qualified doctors found that it was important to land their first post in the team of someone who was good, and who knew all the right people. For when the time came for the young doctor to apply for his next appointment, his consultant could simply pick up the phone on his behalf to secure it. Now that there is a more firmly regulated training programme in place. But in Pappworth's day such programmes were far from the norm. The system worked for you as long as you were able to access help from senior colleagues. That was not the way Pappworth operated.

Pappworth was successful in his first application, to be resident medical officer at the newly-opened Cumberland House Hospital in Mitcham, Surrey. This had about fifty beds for patients with pulmonary tuberculosis who were awaiting transfer to a sanatorium. Pappworth was the only resident member of the medical staff. He was surprised to find that, although the hospital had been opened only recently, it had no facilities for laboratory or X-ray investigations. Pappworth also worked at two other local hospitals, in Epsom and Redhill. He recalls frequent visits to Cumberland House by Dr Patterson, deputy Medical Health Officer of Surrey. 'One day he told me that in view of my qualifications and experience he was surprised that I had accepted the post in Mitcham, but informed me that he presumed I did so because I wanted promotion to a post at St Helier Hospital, Carshalton, which was then in the process of being built. In fact, I knew nothing about that hospital but assured him that that was my intention!' The 800-bed hospital was taken over in 1940 by the government-controlled Emergency Medical Services.

It was during Pappworth's time at Cumberland House that the Second World War broke out and St Helier came so swiftly under the government's wing. Pappworth was invited to become the hospital's first senior resident physician. The previous medical superintendent at Redhill Hospital, who was transferred to St Helier, 'had been very impressed by my diagnostic abilities'. Pappworth felt appreciated and satisfied – for the time being, at least – that he had made it, if not to the heart of the capital, then at least to its outer suburbs. He liked the flat in the hospital provided for him: it had a lounge, dining room, bedroom and bathroom. This may have been the first time in his life that Pappworth was able to relish the privacy and relative luxury of brand-new, purpose-built accommodation. Once again, his memoir records his salary: £600 per annum, with free board and accommodation.

The healer goes into battle

He was not to enjoy these conditions for long. It was natural for him to enter the army and play a part in Britain's fight against Hitler, who had started to spread his anti-Semitic laws across Europe. Pappworth was conscripted in 1941 into the Royal Army Medical Corps (RAMC) with the rank of Second Lieutenant. The requisite training at Aldershot lasted six months. Pappworth 'found the daily parades and drills and marching to the bellowing of a bullying Sergeant Major both boring and sometimes even distasteful, especially when it was entirely irrelevant to any medical duties. Later I was sent on a gas course, which was even worse. We were submitted to many indignities, such as being sprayed from a low-flying aircraft, without prior warning, accompanied by shouts from the officer in charge of "Gas Attack!" Panic-stricken, we tried desperately to don gas masks and gas capes quickly, and our metal helmets. In fact the sprayed liquid was not mustard gas... but merely paint.'

After completing his training, which included lectures laced with 'smutty stories' on tropical medicine and entomology (the scientific study of insects), Pappworth was automatically promoted to Captain. His first posting was a very brief one to York, at the army headquarters of the 56th Infantry Division. Its recruits, including Pappworth, saw service in North Africa and Italy. His regiment was then transferred to Exmouth in Devon. Soon after arrival, Pappworth was asked for help by the senior medical officer of the division, a Brigadier General. He had recently discovered that, only two weeks before the unit was due to go abroad, the regimental medical officers had failed to check the troops' medical categories. Neither had they given them typhoid inoculations. There had been no instruction in first aid or the perils of venereal disease. 'He put me in charge of these activities and, as a reward, he promised to get me posted as Major (medical specialist), for which I had the necessary qualifications and experience.' Pappworth had clearly impressed his superiors with his skills.

In the winter of 1941, he found himself en route for Scotland, travelling by train to Invergordon. From there, he boarded a 'packed boat the size of a Mersey passenger ship', sailing through the night to the small, 100-bed military hospital in Lerwick, on the Shetland Islands. Here, as promised, he was promoted to major. But he had to wait alone for more than three hours before the RAMC colonel 'condescended to see me.'

Pappworth described the colonel and his major as 'pre-war RAMC officers', who were 'both worse for drink' when he first encountered them. Invited to dine with the pair, 'The first question I was asked was how long I had been in the RAMC. When I replied that it was just less than six months, the Major pointed to his three ribbons, generally known as "Pip, Squeak and Wilfred", the three automatic awards after service in the First World War. In no uncertain terms he let me know that he had worked and reached the rank of Major only after twenty years in the RAMC and that, moreover, he considered that they had no need for a specialist in medicine on the Islands. It was the beginning of a very unpleasant stay there.'

I never saw Pappworth's own war medals; maybe he never bothered to claim them. He certainly never wore them when our synagogue held special commemorative services.

As Pappworth confessed, he was 'very miserable' in Lerwick, where he found himself bent almost double as he walked to avoid being blown over by the powerful winds. However, after less than two months, he was posted to 104 British General Hospital in Wiltshire, a medical facility formed to go overseas. Not long afterwards, he found himself on a troop ship in Liverpool, bound for a mystery destination.

North Africa, Italy and Greece: front-line medicine

This turned out to be Algiers. On disembarkation, his company marched for about five miles in the heat to El Arish, carrying large quantities of equipment. Pappworth served in a hospital classified as an 800-bed unit, encamped in tents along the lines of communication between Algiers and the rear forces of the Eighth Army, engaged in a tactical stalemate with Rommel's Panzer Army Africa after the Battles of El Alamein in 1942. 'Very soon we were swamped with casualties.' Most of these were suffering from conditions such as malaria, dysentery, hepatitis and diphtheria. The senior officer, a colonel, agreed to expand the hospital to 1,200 beds, but no extra staff were available. The doctors were provided with no means of transport. Pappworth admits that they felt 'very narked and perhaps even jealous' when they witnessed the soldiers of nearby

6th Armoured Division, who were 'well supplied with transport, which they used to take our nursing staff out on jaunts, including sea bathing.'

While serving at 104 Hospital (which was several times uprooted and moved east as the successes of the Eighth Army continued), Pappworth reported an anti-Semitic incident perpetrated by the head of the surgical unit, Lieutenant-Colonel Kirwan Taylor. He was, as Pappworth reports, 'a consultant physician at St George's, London... On several occasions, when drinking in the crowded officers' mess, he proclaimed for all to hear that, in his view, the war had been started by Jews and was being maintained because of them. I complained to the Colonel about this, pointing out that twenty of the officers were in fact Jews, but he sided with Taylor and there the matter rested. But I was very pleased that one night in the dark when going from the mess to his tent, he fell into the contents of the latrine.'

In the Pappworth Archives at the Wellcome Foundation lies a letter, which he had evidently valued sufficiently to preserve, from Lieutenant-General Leese. A 'Personal Message from the Army Commander,' it reads: 'On the occasion of the Jewish New Year I send to all Jewish soldiers serving in the British, Dominion and Allied formations of the Eighth Army, my good wishes. Jewish soldiers, several thousand of whom are serving in the Eighth Army, have borne their full share in our battles. I hope that the Day of Victory, for which they, with their comrades of this Army, have fought so long and so hard, is now close at hand.'

In early 1944, after the Allied landings at Salerno in September 1943, 104 British General Hospital left North Africa for Naples. Here Pappworth was transferred to the 18th Casualty Clearing Station, initially stationed close to Monte Cassino, and based within the captured Italian army barracks. Treatment here was almost entirely for venereal disease. Pappworth observes that 'Many of the poorer class of Italian women were starving, and turned to prostitution. Years later, after the war, I asked the then head of the RAMC, whom I got to know well – Lieutenant-General Drummond – why he had written in the official history of the army that Naples at that time was suffering from an epidemic described as either typhoid or typhus. His reply was that the disquiet engendered in the families of men serving in Italy at the time would have had marked repercussions if they knew that the epidemic was in fact of a venereal disease. So history is thus falsified.' Pappworth always was impatient when it came to a cover-up of the truth.

At 18 Casualty Clearing Station, Pappworth also tended to troops and civilian personnel wounded during the four assaults by the Allies against the Winter Line held by the Germans and Italians. He recalls in his recorded memoir the intense bombing and shelling of the monastery at Monte Cassino, in particular one raid which fell on a nearby Casualty Clearing Station about a mile ahead of where he was stationed. The Allies suffered terrible casualties after each assault. It was something he never talked about to his family. Another topic about which he, more surprisingly, failed to reminisce was his witnessing of a major natural catastrophe. Pappworth's unit had landed in Italy shortly before the March 1944 eruption of Mount Vesuvius. In his tape-recording, Pappworth describes how 'the whole of the Naples area was... still covered in dense black smoke and ashes'. But he kept to himself the photographs he took and (amazingly, for he was always a great hoarder) allowed them to disappear from his memorabilia.

During his time in North Africa and Italy, Pappworth conducted services every Sabbath. By his own admission, he always had a poor singing voice, but was fortunate to have a private with not only a good voice but also a sound knowledge of Hebrew. The orderly officer in charge of non-officer personnel, Captain Finer, was Jewish, but 'every week I had to plead with him to allow Jewish troops, not only from our own unit but also neighbouring units, to attend our services'.

Pappworth describes with enthusiasm a Seder night (the festive meal marking the start of Passover) that he and Rabbi Berman, the senior Jewish padre in Italy, organised in April 1944. This was celebrated in a large field, twelve miles from Monte Cassino. 'The staging and singing of the famous Haggadah songs were shared out to anyone who wished to sing, either alone or with the rest of us. Never was "Next Year in Jerusalem" sung or shouted with more fervour... A large hospital tent was erected – in fact a whole series of tents – by the Indian Ordinance Unit of the Eighth Army. The tables were large planks covered with hessian, mounted on over one thousand empty petrol drums, all supplied and erected by the Royal Engineers... Over five hundred soldiers attended that marvellous night. We were supplied with matza [unleavened bread], kosher jam and tins of fruit. The eggs were powdered ones: two thousand portions had been obtained by Rabbi Berman on the black market, at ninepence per portion. The Chief Jewish Chaplain of the American Fifth Army supplied fresh butter, tins of tuna fish and fruit juices.'

After the matza baked in Algiers arrived 'very hard and half an inch thick… the American padre came to our rescue and sent us six hundred pounds of a good American matza… We had a selected number of kosher wines… and two hundred litres of local Italian red wine… On order from headquarters, the main roads to the area were blocked so that no vehicles could approach during our Seder.'

This uplifting account of a Jewish festive meal during a war that saw most of Europe's Jewish population destroyed, and a celebration to which non-Jews contributed whole-hearted practical support, offers a moving symbol of hope. That 'marvellous night' was clearly one of the high points of Pappworth's war – and it was one wartime story that he did choose to tell his children. During difficult times throughout his life, Pappworth found solace in his Jewish identity. One aspect of that joyous experience that would have pleased Pappworth immensely was not only the kindness of others, but also their efficiency. Incompetence irritated him, both in his army service and throughout his life.

After the assaults on Monte Cassino, Pappworth travelled to the captured monastery in an 'exciting but frightening journey by trucks up the steep mountain pathways', and then to an encampment a few miles from Rome. He and his unit were allowed to enter the city as tourists, setting up a Casualty Clearing Station about ten miles to the north. After a brief spell, Pappworth was moved to Florence, where his unit was instructed to join the newly-formed 10th Corps – a mixture of British, American and other nationals – and proceed to southeast Italy. The final liberation of the country was anticipated. 'At night we slept under hedges surrounding farms.' He was posted to 98 British General Hospital in Barletta, close to the port of Bari.

By the time Pappworth's work in Italy was completed, the war in Europe was virtually over. But two further RAMC postings were to mean that, for him, war service extended well beyond 1945. He was initially sent to Greece, where British troops assembled as civil war broke out there. Characteristically, Pappworth supported the underdog: 'As usual, the British were supporting the monarchy against the left-wing Greek KKE, who had in fact done most of the fighting against the Germans and the Italians.' He had been instructed to get to Greece as quickly as possible, as there were no experienced British physicians there. The most expeditious way was for Pappworth to be parachuted into the country; fortunately, his objection that he had had no experience of parachuting was accepted. So he avoided a wartime story that might have sounded exciting but would certainly have been a risky venture. He battled to travel to Salonika (Thessaloniki) on a hospital ship, rather than a combat plane.

After the war, Pappworth made a point of reading up on the Jewish community of Salonika: it had been a significant presence in the city since 1492, but had suffered much persecution. When the Germans entered Salonika in April 1941, they requisitioned many Jewish buildings, including the community's hospital, banned Jews from cafés, and confiscated their radios. In the summer of 1942, more than 7,000 Jewish men aged between eighteen and forty-five were enrolled into forced labour. Within ten weeks, twelve percent of these had died.

In return for halting the forced labour, the Germans demanded a ransom equivalent to $40,000, paid in gold. This sum was raised with difficulty by European and American Jews. At the end of that year, the fifteenth-century Jewish cemetery of Salonika was expropriated and used as a quarry. It had contained half a million graves. The gravestones were used to pave streets and latrines. Synagogues and Jewish libraries were raided, their contents sent to Germany. Sixteen of nineteen synagogues were destroyed; the remaining three turned into brothels. The Jews of Salonika were, as elsewhere, forced to wear the yellow armband bearing its Star of David.

Jews were forbidden to use public transport and squeezed into ghettos, their assets seized. On 14 March 1943, the first contingent of Salonika's Jews learned that it was being sent to a new home in Poland: 10,000 people were hounded into railway trucks, permitted one food parcel and fifteen kilograms of additional clothing. From that day onwards, Jews of all ages were marched to the railway station and shipped to Poland. The transports ripped a total of 45,000 Jews, at least ninety-five percent of Salonika's Jewish population, from the city in which their families had lived for generations. All were destined for Auschwitz-Birkenau.

The recent fate of his fellow-Jews in this Greek city had a profound effect on Pappworth. Salonika was re-occupied by the Greek and Allied Forces in October 1944, shortly before his arrival. He found that 'only a handful of Jews remained there. I saw the details of the obscenity of the cemetery headstones used as paving stones.' Here, he came face to face with a tiny part of the evidence that the world was to uncover with the liberation of Europe's concentration camps. The revelation of one of history's greatest acts of systematised evil must have left him speechless with grief. Here was another experience he never discussed with his children.

From Salonika, Pappworth's hospital and its personnel were sent to Volos, a naval base south of Salonika on the way to Athens. The patients suffered various fevers; once at the hospital, they also became distressed by the huge colony of bedbugs thriving behind the wallpaper. One of Pappworth's patients, Dr John McCrae, had also studied medicine at Liverpool. He was to become a close friend, and will be mentioned later for his part in the Pappworth story.

In the spring of 1945, Pappworth attended a Greek Orthodox Easter service at the cathedral in Volos. He was notified that a special Seder night service for Passover would be held in Athens. Members of the Allied forces were especially welcome. With a fellow doctor, Captain Solomons, Pappworth travelled to Athens. His account of this 1945 Seder, although not as exuberant as that makeshift but 'marvellous night' in Italy one year earlier, shows again that an event which connected Pappworth to his Judaism would always be among those memories of war he chose to hold in his mind.

Observant Jews hold two Seder services, on successive evenings. The first Seder night in Athens 'was conducted in the communal hall of the main synagogue. All Jewish civilians, as well as the troops, were invited, and the congregation was large.' The second night 'would be held at the homes of the civilian members'. They would meet the Allied troops at the synagogue and each 'take one or two home with them'. But 'Consternation arose that evening when nobody at all of the civilians turned up to act as hosts. So the padre had to improvise hurriedly a second Seder night, and could not go with the officers – who had been invited to the president's house.'

The 'president' would have been the lay head of the synagogue. Apparently, he and his family were unable to read Hebrew, so the service at his home was conducted by Solomons and Pappworth. The latter failed to persuade his hosts that, after the festive meal, 'there were further portions of the Haggadah to read, including the famous songs'. This is only too credible. Years later, when hosting and leading the Seder service surrounded by his family and friends (some as unfamiliar with Hebrew as his wartime Greek hosts), he insisted on reading virtually every word. He was, in this as in everything he undertook, a rigid perfectionist.

One outcome of the Seder in Athens was that Pappworth met 'a very attractive young woman', whom he invited to dine at a local restaurant prized for its fish. 'She did turn up at the agreed time and place, but was accompanied by her mother, who insisted on coming to dine with us.' Not quite the *rendezvous* he had anticipated.

India: the injuries of class and caste

Shortly afterwards, Pappworth was instructed to return to Bari, where he was granted two weeks' leave in England. The war in Europe was over, but not the Japanese war. Those who had already spent over two years abroad were not eligible for service in the Far East. This rule did not, however, apply to field officers. Many senior officers had already been demobilised, creating a potentially a serious shortage of specialists in all units. So it was that Pappworth found himself posted to India. His impressions of the officers he met on board the Cunard liner, the *Georgic*, led him to observe in his taped memoir: 'I suppose we won the war because many of the German high command were as incompetent as were many of our own senior officers.'

Just a few days before Pappworth landed in Bombay in August 1945, the bombs fell on Hiroshima and Nagasaki. The Japanese surrendered. 'My immediate thought was, how long would it be before I got home?' But he was to stay in India until well after the official end of the Second World War. Bombay greeted him with the extremes of the Indian climate: the monsoon season had started. 'I was fascinated to see police on point duty, standing on high raised platforms, whistles in the mouth ready, and protected from the elements by huge umbrellas. The torrential, incessant downpour was unlike anything I had myself previously experienced.'

Pappworth travelled by train to the famous Red Fort in Delhi, then used as a military barracks. He briefly became a tourist, taking in the Viceroy's Palace, and the Taj Mahal in Agra. Soon afterwards he was moved to 1 British General Hospital in Avadi, near Madras (now Chennai), in south-east India. Recording his memories of this train journey more than forty years later, he recalled that 'The second-class carriages were packed, many standing there through a very long journey. They were surrounded by their luggage, and often had chickens and other birds in baskets... More remarkable was the huge number of those travelling dangerously, seated on the roof of the carriages... I learnt on good information that deaths due to this mode of travel were fairly frequent. Apparently they did this because they had no tickets.'

In charge of the medical division of the large hospital in Avadi, Pappworth initially found himself very busy. He was having to deal with the clinical needs of former British prisoners of war, both military and civil, including POWs from the notorious Burma-Siam railway. Promoted to Lieutenant-Colonel, Pappworth had between 400 and 500 patients arriving daily over a two-week period. His job was to supervise their sorting into three categories: 'those fit enough to be sent to nearby camps awaiting shipping to Blighty; those who, although not seriously ill, required immediate medical attention; and those who were admitted to 1 British General Hospital.' Most of this last group suffered from severe malnutrition and infections, especially malaria, dysentery and hepatitis. Some had unhealed war wounds. 'A tragic group were those who had, as a direct result of malnutrition, become blind because of atrophy of their optic nerves.' About ten former POWs became blind as a result of drinking methylated spirits as an alcohol substitute. 'So, for a few weeks, I was very busy and happily occupied with interesting medical work.'

An added bonus was Pappworth's surprise reunion with fellow Liverpool medical alumnus Stuart Macpherson, Regimental Medical Officer to an East African unit. Gradually, Pappworth began to find that his workload was dwindling, and his thoughts turned still more urgently to the chance of going home. Demobilisation depended on his age and length of service. After about six months in India, his 'number' came up, and so he was entitled to be sent back to England. By then, however, there was a great shortage of well-qualified specialists in southern India, and Brigadier Goldby forbade Pappworth to leave. 'After a year in India,' declares Pappworth, 'I decided on the drastic measure of filling in all the forms myself, including the demobilisation papers and ticket for transport to London. And I got away with it.' He confessed to me how frustrating he had found it to be stranded in India when most other people's lives were returning to something approaching normality. Pappworth travelled home by boat and was granted nearly one year's leave on full pay as Lieutenant-Colonel, 'plus extras for every day spent abroad, which was over four years, the total being well over a thousand pounds.'

Pappworth's observations of extreme poverty and destitution in India, widely apparent on the streets of its major cities, was to have a profound influence on the ethics that informed *Human Guinea Pigs*, and in particular on Pappworth's views on the value of human life and the importance of caring for the sick or injured. During his time in Madras, 'It always appeared to me that Indians, unfortunately including doctors, seemed to value human life so little. It was a common sight to see people lying in the gutters obviously in great distress, many obviously dying, but being unceremoniously ignored by the hordes of passers-by, including doctors.'

He was also horrified by India's caste system, and the racism recounted through an incident at 1 British General Hospital. 'Nearly all the nursing staff were male Indians, and they looked after the wards containing the Africans.' One day he was urgently called to a ward and found an African patient 'being restrained by several hefty British sergeants, because he was trying to kill one of the Indian nurses'. Refused a second helping of the midday meal, this patient had then watched the nurse empty large amount leftover food into a bin. 'So infuriated was he that he set on him, shouting that he was going to kill him, which I believed he was capable of doing. Immediately, though frightened, I decided that the Indian had been in the wrong and ordered the sergeants to put him under arrest.' Twenty years later, the Dr Pappworth who sided with the hungry African rather than the socially superior Indian was to champion the vulnerable patient on the ward against the higher 'caste' of the medical establishment.

Post-war tangles with the old school tie

Pappworth was to describe his 'war saga' as mostly 'very boring and very dull, frequently endured in uncomfortable conditions. The incidents he recorded in his taped memoir he refers to as 'occasional highlights', adding as his final verdict, 'Military life was infuriating'. But his wartime work in the RAMC gave him an enormously useful range of clinical experience. This should have proved a bonus in the advancement of his medical career. However, he admits that, returning to St Helier Hospital after a long holiday, he found his position to be 'difficult'. It had been agreed that all appointments to civilian medical posts during the war were precisely that – for the duration of the war only. A consultant physician from St Thomas' Hospital had been appointed as a part-time consultant at St Helier, doing two half-days a week yet with a larger salary than the £800 per annum Pappworth had been paid when working full-time there. As he explains: 'All medical services were in a state of flux as the National Health Service was being planned. Posts designated Senior Resident Medical Officers and the like were to be abolished, and Consultant Physicians were to take their place. As a consequence, many who had served in the various municipal hospitals, but who had no secure tenure, were in difficulties – unless they could persuade the employing authority to grant them the appropriate consultant status even before the National Health Service started.'

Several doctors working for Surrey County Council were in the same position; they decided to seek employment elsewhere with clear consultant status. Pappworth also applied successfully for various consultant posts. But these were 'all in the less desirable parts of the United Kingdom', so he decided to turn down the job offers. He recalls being invited for interview for a consultant post in 'the large dilapidated former workhouse hospital, with very few facilities, in Burnley, Lancashire. On my way to the interview I stayed in Birkenhead, and Rivkah very sensibly pointed out that it was silly on my part to apply for posts which I did not really want to accept if offered. So I did not, much to the annoyance of the Head of the Lancashire Medical Service, turn up for that interview. I was refused any request for my post at St Helier to be made a permanent full-time consultant one.'

Many of the leading provincial and London hospitals were filled with ex-Forces medical personnel whose appointments, mostly as registrars, were temporary. A few were designated 'trainee consultant posts', one of which Pappworth accepted. It was at the Central Middlesex Hospital in Park Royal, near the A40 leading out of north-west London. He already knew two of the consultant physicians there, neither of whom had served in the Forces but who appeared to have secure tenure because they had both been appointed just before the outbreak of war. One of these, Dr Richard Asher (father of actress Jane Asher), had been declared physically unfit and therefore unable to serve, and Pappworth was informed that his position as registrar had yet to be finalised. The post would be advertised, so if Pappworth took the job of 'trainee consultant', he might stand a chance of being appointed consultant in Asher's place.

One of Pappworth's main duties at the Central Middlesex was to tutor former ex-service doctors – temporary registrars, some of whom were trying to pass the exam for Membership of the Royal College of Physicians. He was also allowed to run a private coaching course each Sunday morning. Meanwhile, the consultant post was advertised, both Asher and Pappworth being shortlisted. When the appointment committee couldn't decide between the two, a second committee was formed, 'but unfortunately Asher got the job. My temporary position there was limited to one year, and when that finished I was in difficulties.' Years later, I remember my father's amusement when his old rival seemed at one point about to become the father-in-law of the most popular young man on the planet, one Paul McCartney.

While Pappworth was working at the Central Middlesex, a vacancy came up at the Whittington Hospital in Highgate for a general physician with an interest in neurology: it seemed the perfect fit. After his interview, as he sat outside the interview room awaiting the result, he heard hoots of laughter within. Later, when he asked one of the interviewers to explain this hilarity, he discovered that the candidate himself was making his interviewers laugh – with him, not at him.

A graduate of Cambridge University and the London Hospital, he was asked why he had taken twelve years to qualify. Much to the committee's amusement, he replied that as an undergraduate he had not taken medicine very seriously, spending much of his time involved in sport and winning Blues in boxing and rowing. 'But,' records Pappworth, 'he had the chutzpah to state that if appointed he would thereafter take medicine extremely seriously and this in fact probably was an important factor in getting him the job.' This story highlights the endless difficulties the brilliant but socially awkward Pappworth knocked against. The man who, as a medical student, had hushed his siblings to silence so that he could sit at the kitchen table and study, found again and again that qualifications and experience weren't enough. Against an Oxford or Cambridge Blue they counted for little.

Following this disappointment, Pappworth went back to Birkenhead to live with A.D. and Rivkah, at the same time conducting private Membership classes for a group of six ex-service doctors at the Liverpool Royal Infirmary. His position was never officially recognised, and he was not allowed to see patients on the wards or in outpatient clinics. Five of his six students passed the Membership of the Royal College of Physicians – an unusually high pass rate, and testament to the high quality of Pappworth's tutoring skills. But 'my position was personally unsatisfactory, as I was treated by the consultants as an outsider'. So Pappworth tasted the bitterness of that 'outsider' status he was to retain for the rest of his career.

When Allan Gaw suggested in his interview with Helen Bamber that Pappworth was always very pre-occupied with the 'Establishment', and also very angry, Bamber readily agreed: 'Oh he was angry. He contained it well, but he was angry'. She added, 'He never swore.'

His next move was to the area of Windsor, Slough and Maidenhead, where he became a consultant physician for five half-days of four hours each. 'I did not enjoy working there very much. Right from the start it was indicated to me that my appointment was not at the request of the local consultants, who felt that they could manage themselves without any extra consultants being appointed.' The main hospital, and the only one of any importance according to the local consultants, was the King Edward Hospital in Windsor. There were already two part-time consultant general physicians on the staff, one of whom, according to Pappworth, 'was regarded as a very boring, dull chap... The other chap had no higher qualifications and only the London conjoint diploma ... no medical degree. He had a private general practice, but was also Medical Officer for Eton School [ie Eton College] and the staff of Windsor Castle. I had a few talks with him mainly concerning medical problems, and his ignorance appeared to me to be unbelievable, but he was tall, attractive-looking... always smartly dressed, and had a very upper-class type of accent.'

This passage reveals Pappworth's conviction, from the start of his career, that he was panting to keep up with men who were his inferiors as doctors. These were the men with the useful social contacts, the tall (unlike him), handsome men who spoke with the right accent, wore the right clothes and had the right connections in the public schools and the aristocracy; the men who for whom Greenway Road, Birkenhead was alien, even incredible territory.

Pappworth concedes that the official neurologist at the King Edward in Windsor, Swithin Meadows, was 'a first-class clinician', also on the staff of two London hospitals: the Westminster and Queen's Square, the latter one of the leading neurological hospitals in the world. 'An interesting point,' observes Pappworth, 'was that he failed on several attempts to obtain a consultant post at Liverpool Royal Infirmary, although he was a Liverpool graduate. But after a long struggle... he finally made it in London.' This, of course, was what Pappworth fully intended to do.

The other Windsor hospital was The Old Windsor. This had been the local workhouse and, remarked Pappworth, 'it still looked like it'. During the war, Nissan huts had been erected as part of the Emergency Medical Service. Though intended to be temporary structures, these remained to house patients for many years afterwards. The hospital had no facilities for pathology or radiology. If these were necessary, the patient had to be referred to the King Edward.

The Old Windsor was essentially a geriatric unit, and a place for the chronically ill. The latter included a group of young people who were 'generally grossly disabled because of various chronic progressive neurological diseases'.

All of them had previously been patients at Queen's Square. The famous neurological hospital, by moving them to Windsor, had according to Pappworth 'stripped themselves of responsibility of further looking after these patients'.

Pappworth's outpatient clinics at the King Edward were, in his words, 'taken from me', and his duties were all transferred to the Old Windsor. The consultant physician there, declared unfit for military service owing to a duodenal ulcer, was the paradigm of a Pappworth poseur: 'Right from the start I was very careful to enquire which patients were his and which were supposed to be under my care. The amazing discovery was that, although [he] had been officially the consultant during and since the war, in fact he had not seen any patients [in Windsor] for several years. He had a few sessions in the West London Hospital, Fulham, and in the Aylesbury Hospital area. So his habit was to drive first to Old Windsor Hospital and there to have a coffee and a short chat with a senior nurse, and then leave without doing any medical work whatsoever there! But he proceeded to drive to Aylesbury to do clinics there. For his visits to Old Windsor Hospital, he was paid for half a day's work.'

The point of Pappworth's story is not that he felt personally disgruntled, but that he was incensed by the way patients (and, for that matter, the finances of the recently-created NHS) were being badly let down by the indolence of a particular doctor. During this period Pappworth also worked in Slough, doing two sessions: one outpatient and one for inpatients. He describes the hospital as 'an old large decrepit workhouse, which over ten years later was demolished and a brand new hospital, Wexham Park, was built'. A state-of-the-art new hospital had been badly needed in Slough, as the town's population expanded. Another colleague gave Pappworth further proof of the casual work ethic shown by some senior doctors. This doctor, who also had a few sessions at the West London Hospital in Fulham and at the Hammersmith Hospital, worked two official sessions in Slough.

Pappworth takes up the story: 'Soon after my first visit to that hospital I met [him] and asked him which beds and therefore which patients were under his care, and which were to be under my care. His immediate, amazing reply was "Pappworth, you have all of them!" His outpatient work was equally surprising. All the patients, both new and old, were seen by a recently qualified doctor or a slightly more senior doctor who had no higher qualifications. [He] came along towards the end of the outpatients' session and read the notes which had been made on the patients seen the previous week, and he accepted the clinical findings and noted the results of any investigations, which that junior staff had previously ordered. He then dictated a letter to the patient's GP as though he had been in complete control of the patient from the outset. Few of those he in fact he himself saw. He very rarely bothered to go into any of the wards. For this he received payment for two sessions per week.'

This recollection could be dismissed as Pappworth bleating, in which he exposes the incompetence, dishonesty even, of a former colleague. But it is significant that during these twenty or so years between his discharge from military service and the publication of *Human Guinea Pigs*, Pappworth was watching, noting, gathering a sense of what it means to be a good doctor who puts the patient's needs first – and what, in British medical practice, was foul and in need of a public washing.

Still working on the Berkshire/Buckinghamshire border, Pappworth was given a regular session at the old workhouse hospital in Maidenhead, which had more than four hundred beds but no laboratory or X-ray facilities. Once again, we find him experiencing a medical institution that cried out for improvement. The hospital consisted of a series of two or three-storey blocks, and 'the approach above ground floor was by very worn stone steps up winding staircases which were very difficult for stretchers to pass. There were no lifts.' Some time later, when Pappworth was a consultant locum at St George's in east London, he found himself once again working in a dilapidated building, badly hit during the Blitz. Under the floorboards lurked wild cats. Helen Bamber, a social worker there at the time, recalled the efforts of those 'courageous doctors... The docks were dying, there was a lot of unrest in Wapping; it was quite a volatile area. There were a lot of lot of accidents in the docks,' and 'We had more and more people trundled in with... the most appalling injuries.' Pappworth was dealing with that wide range of emergency conditions which was to contribute to his unparalleled expertise as a general physician.

At the old workhouse hospital in Maidenhead, the patients were officially cared for by two local GPs, who consulted Pappworth by phone or note but very rarely met with him. 'Two groups of patients especially shocked me. Firstly, a large number of old people with fractured thigh-bones... who had been bedridden ever since their initial injury and had never seen an orthopaedic surgeon, and surgery on them had never been even considered. The other group was one of geriatric patients who had enlarged prostates but had never been operated on, and had been left with the insertion of a permanent catheter into their bladder.

With great difficulty I persuaded a local orthopaedic surgeon and general surgeon… interested in prostate surgery to come out to the hospital and transfer some of those to the neighbourhood hospitals where those surgeons were consultants. I had become unofficially a geriatrician.'

One justification for pushing the responsibility for the elderly solely onto Pappworth was the size of the waiting list: over a hundred for geriatric and chronically sick patients. Pappworth found that the only established way these patients had been seen even as outpatients was for GPs to arrange a consultant home visit, for which the consultant was paid a fee. The patient would then get placed on a waiting list for admission to hospital, if this was considered necessary. Pappworth arranged to see all of them at his outpatient clinic, and was 'amazed to find that most of them could be dealt with there and then by me, and there was no need for them to be admitted to hospital at all'. For most of those who did require hospital attention, Pappworth was able to arrange this immediately at the Old Windsor.

So he succeeded in reducing the waiting list to a very few. Pappworth notes that 'the other consultant physicians did not like this, because I had removed from them a source of income, namely domiciliary visits.' He adds, not without a dash of pride, 'I am certain that I was never popular with any of the other consultants.' Pappworth was already set on a path of conflict with his colleagues that, arguably, was integral to his decision to write *Human Guinea Pigs*.

One example of Pappworth's brush with authority was to occur later in the 1950s, as recounted by Helen Bamber in interview with Allan Gaw. While working at St George's in Wapping, Pappworth, along with his colleague John Rundle and a doctor from South Africa, agreed that it would be of great benefit to the patients if the three of them were to hold a monthly clinical meeting that all doctors were welcome to attend. This was an attempt to reach 'a level of proficiency and sophistication' which, according to Bamber, they achieved in a 'really quite remarkable' way.

She describes how 'The doctors began to come monthly, so you would get all the doctors from the locality coming and meeting to discuss with the doctors in the hospital and amongst themselves their patients. Now, what could be better than that?… There were other consultants in the hospital who did not like this at all'. neither did the hospital director like it, 'So, he had enemies wherever he went'.

This tendency to stick to what he believed in certainly didn't help when it came to what we now refer to as networking. When he first started working in the Berkshire/Buckinghamshire area, Pappworth was on several occasions invited to have drinks with his fellow doctors in one of the well-known bars or restaurants. 'But their talk bored me because it dealt mainly with local gossip, especially who was sleeping with whom, and what was happening to "the Windsor Castle set", as some of the locals and a few doctors were labelled. It was all outside my own interests.' Pappworth tried using these social gatherings as a way to obtain more working sessions in the area, or return to looking after patients at the King Edward Hospital, but to no avail.

As always, it was a matter of temperament, personality and even class. He never acquired the social skills to turn the small talk he despised to good account. As Helen Bamber was to explain, it became clear to her that 'people did not like [Pappworth] very much – he was boycotted to a certain extent... [perhaps because of] his outspokenness, his Jewishness, whatever... Also he was uncompromising – and he would not play the game. He really would never play the game... He never conceded to the social patterns and norms of that time – with a drink in one hand and rather sarcastic remarks about colleagues. He would never do that... He was an outsider.'

He simply wasn't prepared to undertake all the political manoeuvring needed to make one's way in hospital medicine. One prejudice of Pappworth's that did him no favours was his dislike of committees. This prevented him from edging into the inner circle. For Pappworth, being a good doctor was above all about looking after your patients, and also training students to become first-class clinicians. It had nothing to do with sitting round a table listening to colleagues discuss policies, finances or paint-colours. But his presence at such meetings would certainly have helped him.

London life for 'the doctor's doctor': marriage, children, independence

Having worked in Windsor, Slough and Maidenhead hospitals for two years, Pappworth resolved it was time to move on. The chief reason for this decision, he claims, was 'an increasing strain because of motoring to the Windsor area [from London], which meant travelling during the rush hours both there and back. I was doing over 30,000 miles per year, mainly for visits to the hospital area, and, in winter, fog was often present very heavily, especially in the low-lying Thames area.' He did not regret his departure. Because he had been working at these hospitals only part-time, he had decided to rent consulting rooms at

66 Harley Street. Here Pappworth could see patients referred to him by GPs. He was gaining a reputation as a brilliant diagnostician, and has been referred to as 'the doctors' doctor'. So, increasingly, he was being asked to diagnose illnesses where his colleagues were unable to do so. They sent members of their family to him. However much Pappworth had made himself *persona non grata* within the medical establishment, colleagues had a deep trust in his diagnostic skills.

GPs working in Belgravia and Mayfair undoubtedly helped him to build up his private practice. One of these, Dr John McRae, who had a large private practice in these affluent parts of London, became a lifelong personal friend, and wrote a letter to the medical press strongly supporting *Human Guinea Pigs* on its publication. Another key ally, who also became one of Pappworth's closest friends, was Dr Stuart Macpherson, with whom Pappworth had enjoyed a re-union in India. He had developed a very large practice in Kuala Lumpur, his patients including government ministers and members of the royal family there. Macpherson sent Pappworth VIPs from Malaysia, which is how the latter developed a close association with the Far East – including also Singapore and Hong Kong. Stuart Macpherson and his Chinese Malaysian wife May moved back to the UK on his retirement, choosing to live in a block of flats a few minutes up the hill from Pappworth's home.

While working in Windsor, Pappworth had been living in London in the White House, Albany Street, near Regents Park. This consisted of bachelor flats, and also contained a 'fairly good restaurant, which I often used', a swimming pool and a squash court. He then lived for a time with his friend Sidney Nathan (later to be Pappworth's best man) and his wife Hilda, at 1 Frognal Gardens in Hampstead. He then moved to number 2, renting a bedroom in the flat of another Hilda – Popper – and her husband, refugees from Czechoslovakia. Their one child, Tula, was away at boarding school. Most of Pappworth's meals were eaten with the Poppers, and he grew very fond of the family. Sadly, Popper died of lung cancer after a short illness, whereupon Hilda decided to emigrate with Tula to Israel, where her only surviving relatives lived. I remember visiting Hilda and Tula at their home in Haifa in 1965. Their affection for Maurice was very evident: it's not often that I recall my father happily submitting to a warm hug and embrace.

It was while living at the White House that Pappworth himself became the patient, suffering a severe bout of renal colic which left him 'in agony'. Since early childhood he had never been ill. Now he was at the receiving end, and had great difficulty in contacting a GP for a home visit. Eventually, after several hours of severe pain, Pappworth was injected with morphine by one Dr Finch of Golders Green. By the following day he was already feeling well. An X-ray showed a stone in the lower end of the ureter near its opening into the bladder; a later X-ray indicated that it had not budged. This second X-ray, a specialist one called an intravenous pyelogram, revealed a mild degree of damage to one of Pappworth's kidneys. But, if the stone were removed, this damage would be only temporary. Pappworth consulted Mr Ferguson of the Central Middlesex, a surgeon who specialised in such conditions, and was admitted to that hospital, where the stone was successfully removed.

There was a small possibility that drinking a lot of fluid would dislodge the stone. So late December 1952 saw Maurice Pappworth imbibing large quantities of beer in the company of Sidney and Hilda Nathan. The therapy took place at the home of the Nathans' friends Harry and Trudy Sacker, who at the time lived near Harrow. Harry Sacker was the first of the significant new people to enter Pappworth's life as he awaited surgery. They were to remain lifelong friends, Sacker becoming (as we shall see) his lawyer.

The second – and more important – acquaintance was made on the same evening. Several pints in, Hilda Nathan suggested that Maurice go to an exhibition she had arranged of paintings by Archie Ziegler at a private house in Highgate. Maurice duly went along, and purchased for £40 an oil landscape of Céret, a town in southern France in the Pyrenees. Apparently it hung in the hall of the family home, but I must admit to having no recollection of it. It was at this exhibition that Maurice first met and was introduced to Jean Goldberg, the woman who was to become his wife. (She, incidentally, never liked that painting of Céret.) According to her version of events, Maurice kept on approaching her, bottle in hand, with the words 'More wine, Jeanie?'

Her parents being in South Africa at the time, she was staying at the home of their friends Dr Henry and Winnie Lewis on the Finchley Road. Their son, Kenneth, was to become our family doctor: we always referred to him as 'Dr Kenneth'. That evening, Maurice gave Jean a lift back to the Lewises, and she then visited him when he was at the Central Middlesex for his operation. They became engaged in April 1953 (he proposed, she claims, over a plate of sausages) and were married at Maurice's synagogue, the Western, on 4 October 1953, by Rabbi David Miller.

They had known one another for less than a year, but at the time of his wedding Maurice was forty-three, and Jean was thirty – at that time considered almost 'over the hill' for a woman. I remember her annoyance when, with the tactlessness of childhood, I once exclaimed, 'Goodness, Mum! I've just realised Dad's closer in age to Granny and Grandpa [her parents] than to you.' They both desperately wanted children, and I suspect this may have been one of the chief drivers of their marriage.

Our father remained characteristically circumspect about his earlier liaisons, whereas our mother was happy to regale us with stories of her past boyfriends. They included a marquis, a penniless artist who borrowed money from her with which to buy her bunches of flowers, and the former fiance who broke off the engagement when she was living in a caravan and suffering from the effects of a bee sting on her eye. Her parents, who lived in Davies Street, Mayfair, were from the kind of affluent background in which Maurice never would have dreamed of gaining a foothold. Jean's father, Philip Goldberg, had started his career in the family furniture business (his younger brother Geoffrey disgraced himself by running off with one of the models who reclined on their sofas in advertisements), and then took over the highly successful Town and City Properties.

The newly-weds spent their wedding night at Brown's Hotel in London, and honeymooned in Florence. Their first home was in Keats Close, a group of six houses next to Keats House in Hampstead, experimentally created during the 1930s for those who valued a sense of community above privacy. There were no hedges or fences between the gardens. Jean and Maurice both loved the house, and he must have felt great pride in being able to provide such a pleasant married home for his bride. But he was all too aware of the need to increase his income. 'During the period of our engagement, and indeed even after we were married, my medical career was in a state of flux and great uncertainty. But Jean never appeared to be in the least interested about my career' and its difficulties. In this she was reproducing the attitude of her own mother, who seems to have remained firmly detached from the business skills Philip exerted to ensure a very comfortable lifestyle for his wife.

A New Generation

Maurice and Jean wasted no time. I am the eldest of their three daughters, and I was born (a week late) exactly ten months after their wedding day. My mother whispered to me that I was named Joanna after Anna Freud. But that is something she would not have admitted to her anti-Freudian new husband. He arranged an X-ray, so that they could both see *in utero* their eagerly awaited infant. This was, surely, a risky and surprising move.

After my birth at St Mary's Paddington, the proud father sat stolidly next to his wife's bed while she breast-fed me, deaf to the midwives' insistence that this was contrary to the rules. My sister Dinah was born twenty months later, and Sara two years after that. There is no doubt that Maurice would have liked a son. But Jean, the older of two daughters, decided that three was enough. Years later, she declared that 'your father would have had such high expectations of him.'

Maurice certainly enjoyed having daughters. I remember him taking me into town and buying me my perfect dress – white and frilly, with a sticking-out petticoat and a print of sprinkled rosebuds. My mother didn't approve. As a small child my sister Dinah, who looked very like our father, had beautiful long blonde ringlets. When, at the age of eight, she had her hair cropped short at his wife's instigation, Maurice was seriously displeased. But he hated to think that any of us was making the slightest attempt to lure the opposite sex, and made clear his dislike of heavy make-up. In this his attitude resembled that of his father, who raised those six unmarried daughters.

When it came to education, he was ambitious for his three daughters. He helped me to understand his beloved chemistry, and wrote to the headmistress to complain when Dinah was sent out at the start of her O level physics exam because (like her father, never afraid to cause fuss) she'd exclaimed volubly at the quality of her desk. Reluctant to talk about medicine at home, he never encouraged us to consider studying the subject. When at the age of twenty-nine Dinah decided to switch her career from town planning to midwifery, friends and family cried to her 'But your father was a doctor; you went to Cambridge! You should become a doctor too'. Perhaps Maurice Pappworth had put off his very clever middle daughter from following in his footsteps.

One of the reasons he was so pleased Dinah studied at Cambridge and I at Oxford was that he understood how a degree from those universities would open for us doors he had found closed against him. We would have the right kind of pedigree. Pappworth was in many ways very conventional in his views on education, distrusting (as with the teaching of medicine) anything that smacked of the inauthentic. His pleasure in my love of literature, and my decision to pursue it at university, may lie partly in childhood memories of those poetry sessions with his adored sister Rivkah – rare moments of boyhood intimacy with a family member.

We all loved the house in Keats Close, where our father photographed us in the garden playing at being nurses (never doctors), or cowgirls, and enjoying the slide which converted into a seesaw. The most exciting room was the attic, which our father had converted into his own personal sanctuary. As in his childhood, when he and A.D. had developed their hobby in the basement of Greenway Road, Maurice created a dark room. There he developed and printed the black-and-white photos he took on his Rolliflex. It seemed such a privilege to climb the ladder up to his secret place. I am trying now to make its pungently acidic smell remind me of times spent close to my father. When we moved house to the Vale of Health in July 1961, one of the three bathrooms was pressed into service as a dark room, its tightly-fitted blinds left permanently closed. Dinah, whose bedroom was just along the corridor, felt comforted by the gentle night-time sounds emanating from it, which included our father's 'occasional spirited off-key rendition of "Oseh Shalom"' (meaning 'Bring Peace', this sung verse concludes a number of important Jewish prayers'.

Our father also took up the movie camera with great enthusiasm. Family holidays occurred at Christmas. During the summer our mother normally hired a cottage with friends, and the female Pappworths would troop off to Suffolk, Cornwall or Wales, leaving Maurice to the large old house in the Vale of Health on the edge of Hampstead Heath, and to the running of his courses.

Our parents were quite pioneering in their choice of regular Christmas and New Year destination. Only a few Brits went skiing in the 1960s. Among these intrepid foreigners on the slopes of the Swiss Alps were the diminutive Pappworths, struggling with the enormous skis of those days, the cold air scarcely warded off by woollen ear-warmers knitted by Auntie Esther. Our parents didn't ski: they walked in the mountains, from which our father would occasionally sprout up before us. He stood there with, as our mother put it, 'a camera dangling from every branch of his anatomy'. Back in England, we would sit in front of our father's screen and watch ourselves on nursery slope and piste, our technical solecisms all too glaring. More enjoyable to watch were the children's birthday parties, which our father always made a point of filming. The fancy dress ones were the best, along with the scene featuring the three of us dressed up as characters from the Purim story. We won first prize in the synagogue's competition.

Our father loved having small children though, as often happens, the relationship became more complicated as we grew older and wriggled out from under that uncompromising paternal shadow. He taught us to play chess: as I grew older, and the games between us more serious, he would sacrifice his queen at the beginning to give me a head-start. As with Naomi when she was very small, he told us stories.

There were three recurring tales, the first featuring Mary and Judith (fairly obvious representations of Dinah and me – the naughty and the good), the second Pimpernotta and Scratchibaldi, both irredeemably naughty and later to make a reappearance as theoretical types in Pappworth's last medical book, and finally our beloved Roomo Rhino. I think at one point that we really did believe that our father had, in his youth, driven around Merseyside with the family's pet rhinoceros sitting on the roof of the car doing its knitting. He enjoyed inventing characters and slightly ludicrous narrative riffs, and these have stayed with me. They offer a certain insight into his success as a teacher.

One particular childhood memory of my father is, like the early sessions in the dark room, special because it was one shared by just the two of us. Every Friday Maurice would stop off at Camden Market on his way home from work; occasionally he took me with him. It was the old street market, with vendors chanting their wares. My father would head with his basket straight for the fruit stall he knew best, where the holder would always greet him as 'Dr Pappworth', make recommendations and offer good deals. It being the Sabbath eve, Erev Shabbat, he would buy a bunch of flowers for Jean and return home in cheerful mood. This was sometimes spoiled; at other times not. At dinner-time she lit the candles; he blessed the wine, the challah, his daughters and – when he felt she deserved it – his wife, with the 'Ayshet Chayil' prayer from the Book of Proverbs. Grace after meals could be a long-drawn-out affair, especially after Dinah started going to a Zionist youth group and taught us how to sing it all, and where to add more songs.

On a Saturday morning, the three girls normally walked with their observant father to and from synagogue, the West Hampstead: up to the top of the Heath, down Frognal, across the Finchley Road and onto West End Lane. It was a long climb back home, but we talked non-stop all the way. We often paused to admire a particularly attractive garden. On one occasion the householder was there, working in the garden, and our father complimented him. Smiling, the man replied, 'Yes, I notice you pass every Saturday. You always strike me – all of you – as particularly happy.' Rather less happy was the time

when Maurice, following the Bible's instructions on the importance of hospitality towards strangers, invited home for lunch with us a man who had visited
the synagogue that morning for the Shabbat service. Jean made it clear to all
that this unexpected extra guest was a source of deep annoyance.

Despite his deep-rooted objections to psychoanalysis, Maurice did allow
his three daughters to attend a nursery school that flourished in the basement of
Maresfield Gardens and close to Sigmund Freud's house (occupied after his
death by Anna, and now the Freud Museum). Our mother claims that he was
very impressed when he visited it. It concentrated on developing social skills,
arts and crafts, music and dance, a love of books... and baking. That is a mad-
eleine memory from my childhood – the smell of biscuits in the oven. For me
it sums up the Freud nursery school, along with its wonderful garden which
offered a child's dream of outdoor play equipment. Maurice later quarrelled
with Manna Friedmann, the widowed German refugee who ran the school. He
believed she was a malign influence on his marriage, who encouraged Jean to
continue in psychoanalysis and thus, as he saw it, drove a wedge between them.
I remember her once in tears in our garden.

Marrying Jean had meant that Maurice suddenly found himself part of a
very different family from his own. Part of what attracted him to her was that
she herself was something of a rebel against her privileged background. They
had met at a party in Hampstead, and it was to the area's leafy promise that,
like her husband, she wished to return after life in Mayfair. At the time when
he first met his new son-in-law, Philip Jonas Goldberg had quite recently sold
his father's firm to Great Universal Stores. The family company included
Smarts Furniture Stores and Boyds Shops, the latter selling pianos and other
musical instruments. Smarts in particular was a thriving organisation, with out-
lets nationwide. With the proceeds of the sale, Philip set up a property company
called Camden City, later changing the name of the growing business to Town
and City Properties.

Goldberg Senior, who had already died when Maurice married Jean, was at
one stage President of the St John's Wood Synagogue. But his son Philip retained a fairly tenuous connection with Judaism. When Maurice visited him and
his wife, Lovie, he had to be treated as a vegetarian, as they didn't keep a kosher
kitchen. They were, however, members of the West London Synagogue: the
flagship of British Reform Judaism, near Marble Arch. Maurice branded Lovie
and Philip 'right-wing Tories' and also anti-Zionists. They had been to Palestine once (in 1926) to visit the grave of Philip's paternal grandfather, buried on

the Mount of Olives, but swiftly fled when a minor earthquake occurred. They returned very briefly to the newly-created state of Israel to persuade their independent-minded older daughter to come back with them to England. Jean had joined the Zionist youth group Habonim, and had gone out to Israel soon after independence in 1948. She loved the country, and had many friends there. This enthusiasm for newborn Israel, and for its high-minded dreams, was perhaps one of the chief differences between Jean and her parents – and one of the things Maurice most liked about her. Later, he discovered that her interest in Israel and her determination to be different from her own mother did not extend to joyous fervour at the prospect of running a kosher, Sabbath-observing household.

Lovie's family, their surname anglicised to 'Bertish', traded in high-quality men's linen and owned Tern Shirts. Her nephew, Cecil Woodburn-Bamberger, entertained Maurice at his large house on Hampstead Lane after the latter's engagement to his cousin. He laced Maurice's requested soft drinks with gin, so that his guest was too intoxicated to drive home and slept in the car until he had sobered up. 'Just testing you out, old boy,' Cecil later admitted to him. Here was an unsettling initiation rite for the working-class northerner about to enter a wealthy London-centred family with roots in South Africa and Rhodesia – alongside distinctly racist opinions. For Maurice, his some of fiancée's relatives belonged to just the type of assimilated Jew he despised. He had a nasty Yiddish word for the specimen: a 'schmatteryid' (rubbish Jew).

Philip Goldberg himself was educated at St Paul's School in London, but his intelligence resided in non-academic areas. Maurice, naturally, noted the fact that his father-in-law failed his matriculation examination. Philip was conscripted into the army as a teenager during the First World War, but was invalided out of France with shell-shock. Throughout his life, Philip appears to have suffered from what Maurice diagnosed as 'occasional bouts of reactive depression, by which is meant a depression of a known emotional cause'. Philip recompensed his son-in-law for informal consultations on his illness in a variety of ways, all of which indicate both imagination and a personal engagement with the family. They ranged from a drawing by Felix Topolski of the Israeli leader Ben Gurion to a bust of his granddaughters for the garden and the funds to buy them a piano. It appears that much of Philip's 'reactive depression' arose from a lack of intimate love in his marriage. Sadly, both his daughters followed in his footsteps by failing to achieve this with their spouses.

Philip seems to have made every effort to welcome Maurice into the family fold. Maurice certainly enjoyed a much warmer relationship with him than with Lovie, who invited me to lunch shortly before my wedding and told me that, if my father spoke at the reception, she simply wouldn't attend. She was convinced he had a chip on his shoulder because of his height, and informed me that he was obsessed with money. Born with the proverbial silver spoon in her mouth, she was possibly not in a position to make an empathetic judgement.

Lovie and Philip were heavy smokers. When Philip was in his late sixties, his GP asked Maurice to look at a spinal X-ray which showed changes typical of cancer secondaries from a primary infection of the chest. Maurice arranged for his father-in-law to be treated by a former student at the Royal Marsden Hospital. Radiotherapy helped significantly to decrease the size of the tumour, but it never disappeared.

In 1969, soon after Philip had completed this radiotherapy, Lovie travelled to the Wrightington Hospital near Wigan for a pioneering type of hip replacement. Philip and Jean accompanied her in the private ambulance that took her north, and stayed at a hotel in Manchester. The following day Maurice received a phone call from Jean: her father had had an epileptic fit, followed by what Maurice describes as 'transient weakness of his right upper lip'. He contacted a friend of his, a former consultant physician in Manchester, who saw Philip and also Lovie as she awaited surgery. She didn't wish this to be postponed. 'Jean was very upset,' records Maurice.

He persuaded his father-in-law to return to London with him. Maurice arranged for him to be seen by a neurologist who agreed with his diagnosis: Philip's lung cancer had metastasised via the spine to his brain. By this time, he was unable to speak. I remember visiting him for the last time: he gave Dinah and me elastic bands encrusted with 'pearls' and sparkling 'crystals' for our hair, which at that time we kept in bunches. I was fifteen. I knew he was dying. Philip passed away at the end of January 1969, two months short of his seventy-first birthday. Maurice claimed that his death lost him a chief ally in the difficulties he was experiencing in his marriage. He turned down the silver swizzle-stick Lovie offered as a memento, but gladly accepted his late father-in-law's gold watch. I have it still.

Chapter Four

Guru and showman: a great teacher at work

'His teaching was like nothing I had before or since: it was like going to the theatre.'

(Dr Pat Broad, former student of Maurice Pappworth)

Maestro of the MCRP

After his marriage, Pappworth worked one afternoon a week at the Leavesden Hospital, near Watford, one of the largest hospitals for 'mental deficients' (as he called them) in the UK. When the Medical Superintendent of Leavesden left to take up a similar position at the Horton Mental Hospital near Epsom, he asked Pappworth to join him there, which the latter was pleased to do. Two of Pappworth's former students were consultants at Horton, which contained the world's largest centre for the treatment of neurosyphilis: a disease Pappworth had quite frequently come across when working in Liverpool. One of the junior staff there was Dr Nina Myer, 'who was regarded by the consultants as a silly woman... They were very pleased that she got a job elsewhere.' She was to play a part in Jean and Maurice's contentious marriage, when many years later she became Jean's psychoanalyst.

Pappworth at this stage was working all over London and the Home Counties. In addition to his job in Watford, he did one session a week at St John's Hospital, a large geriatric institution in Battersea. Again, he encountered a former student in a senior position – in this case as Medical Superintendent. Once a week he worked a session at Friern Barnet, a mental hospital in north London. Attending to the medical needs of the elderly and mentally ill, Pappworth was doing the kind of work which, one suspects, other doctors were often unwilling to take on. As he remarks, his motivation was not wholly altruistic: 'I did this because each of them [these hospitals] had a wealth of clinical material, including conditions rarely seen outside such institutions, and thereby enlarging my own clinical experience, especially of comparatively rare conditions.' Possibly at this stage, Pappworth was able to add some of the particularly arresting images in his collection of medical photographs.

The visits offered a further advantage. He was usually able to take on his hospital visits four or five of his MRCP students, 'who, with the co-operation of the staff and the patients themselves, were allowed to examine selective patients and to be quizzed by me about them. At the request of the medical staff, I gave my opinion on cases with diagnostic problems and helped the running of those hospitals by persuading some of my students to do locums there. Any of the junior staff who co-operated with me, especially in the selection of patients suitable for teaching, I allowed to come to any of my classes they wished to attend without charge'.

The courses that Pappworth ran for thirty years, coaching postgraduates for the Membership of the Royal College of Physicians examination, were to be one of the great successes of his life – and also a means by which he was prompted to write *Human Guinea Pigs*. During the early 1950s he had started to run his classes, having identified a gap in the market. Given the exam's low pass rate and the urgent need of junior and higher-ranking doctors for extra coaching to prepare for this critical hurdle, it struck him as remarkable that there was so little on offer.

Pappworth's classes were held on four evenings a week from 1952 until 1968, and then once a week from 1969, in three successive locations. They immediately became very popular. Classes took place from 5pm until 7.30pm or later, at the end of a working day that for Pappworth had started at 9am and finished only half an hour before the evening class was due to begin. Aspiring young doctors recommended the course to one another. Or if they weren't tipped off by word of mouth, they might have spotted Pappworth's tiny box advertisement in a medical journal. Some were drawn to his MRCP course after reading his *Primer of Medicine*. One radiology registrar was advised that if he wanted to pass the MRCP he should go to Pappworth's classes: 'He's a horrible man,' was the message, 'but he'll get you through the exam.'

When Helen Bamber was helping Pappworth in his research for *Human Guinea Pigs*, he suggested that she attend the classes free of charge, so that she could feel more engaged in the project. Even if they didn't attend a full course, doctors made a point of going to hear him lecture, so that they could listen to somebody who was, according to Professor Martin Gore, 'a household name'. A further attraction was the chance to witness this iconoclast being 'very noisy' on the topic of the medical establishment.

During the 1950s many Australians, New Zealanders and South Africans came to the UK for postgraduate study, and the vast majority of those who wished to become Members of the Royal College of Physicians attended Pappworth's courses. Like the British doctors, many booked places as a result of personal recommendation. It was these overseas doctors who formed the core of his early classes. While later claiming that most of them would have passed without his help, Pappworth noted at the time that, for obvious reasons, these visitors were always keen to pass the exam at the first attempt. Later, Pappworth taught a large number of Asian students.

He resented the accusation that he was chiefly reliant on foreign students, who never formed more than a third of his cohort. More significant, according to his memoirs, was the fact that 'many of my students were... registrars and senior housemen in the various London teaching hospitals, who found that they did not have any genuine postgraduate training in their own hospitals except as future narrow specialists.' Pappworth was also proud of the fact that many of his students came from outside London – from Manchester, Leeds, Birmingham and even the Scottish universities. They would come down for the day specifically to attend his class.

At the beginning of each three-month course, Pappworth capped the number of students at fifty. The students had to be accommodated in the consulting room Pappworth rented on the ground floor of 66 Harley Street, so he divided them into two groups, allowing a maximum of twenty-five at the two duplicate sessions. At these first classes no chairs were available, so the students would sit on the floor. As they left at the end of the evening, they would leave a pound note on the table. This later rose to five pounds, according to the accounts of those who attended his Seymour Hall course. So drained were they by the end of the two-hour session, the doctors rarely socialised afterwards.

I can remember my father's Harley Street consulting room, which I visited only rarely (though he often gave us a lift to school, which was *en route*). Entered through a heavy mahogany door, this imposing but cold and rather untidy space, littered with work in progress, was not unlike the ante-room of a shabby gentlemen's club. On one side a set of curtains screened off the examination couch; straight ahead, the room was dominated by a large, traditional desk and decorated with photographs of his children. He shifted these when he made television appearances from the consulting room, ensuring that his brood was visible beside him. So here was a place that radically re-invented itself for his teaching. The consulting room metamorphosed into something much more informal, with the chairless students sitting, literally, at their master's feet.

The furniture and carpets – not in especially good condition – were provided by Pappworth's landlord at number 66, a gynaecologist who charged extra for these supposedly valuable antiques on top of the rent. After a few years, Pappworth asked if he could replace them with his own furniture, and so reduce his payments as the rent had steadily increased. The landlord objected, and Pappworth, with the help of his solicitor and friend Harry Sacker, found the dispute eventually resolved in his favour. But more trouble was to follow. What Pappworth termed the 'super-landlords', Howard de Walden Estates, which controlled the tenancies of 'all the better consulting rooms in the Harley Street and Wimpole Street area', sent him a letter. It had come to their notice that he was using his consulting room for teaching, which he was not entitled to do under the terms of his lease; he must stop the classes immediately. Pappworth subsequently discovered, without surprise, that his betrayer was the gynaecological landlord with the 'antique' furniture collection.

Pappworth now experienced great difficulty in finding suitable accommodation for his courses. When he mentioned this to his father-in-law Philip, the latter introduced him to the owner of a building on Park Lane due to be demolished in a few months' time to make way for the Bunny Club. In fact, although the arrangement was only temporary, he found the place ideal for his lectures, though expensive to rent.

The Royal College of Physicians would not allow him to use their premises, because his MRCP courses were 'unofficial'. He had no better luck with the Royal Army Medical Centre on Millbank. These premises had seemed like a distinct possibility, as the Lieutenant General of the Royal Army Medical Corps required that all regular army medical officers under his command who wished to be recognised as specialists should attend Pappworth's courses, for which the RAMC paid. Unfortunately, the War Office refused to allow the Millbank building to be used on the grounds that it would mean visits from 'non-military personnel' – in other words, the students.

Maurice continues the story with his usual eye for the humorous: 'Suitable premises had not been found and time was running out before the beginning of my next course. But I had the luck to need the use of the gents' toilet at Oxford Circus, where I saw a large notice advertising premises at Seymour Hall.' Thus, as Pappworth quips in his 1980 article for *World Medicine* on postgraduate exams, he was 'doubly relieved'.

This building, in Seymour Place, belonged to Westminster Council. It had a large swimming pool and has now been turned into a fitness centre. Its manager agreed with the relevant council authority that Pappworth should be allowed to hire a suitable room on the premises. 'This turned out to be an excellent arrangement, and the rent was very modest. The staff were always extremely helpful during the several years I went there until my illness in July 1981.' He says no more about the illness, but we will return to it in the final chapters.

At the master's feet

Classes at Seymour Hall, like those in Harley Street, took place in the evening after work, and lasted at least two hours. Dr Martin Scurr, for example, who attended the course at Seymour Hall during 1975, recalls going to Seymour Hall every week, on a Tuesday or Wednesday evening. His fellow-students were mostly but not exclusively junior hospital doctors. It was all very *ad hoc*. Even when classes were still taking place at Seymour Hall, students usually sat on the floor. There was no secretary who took bookings for the classes: Pappworth handled the administration himself, and payment was by cash only on the day. A single course consisted of a series of eight lectures, and there can be little doubt that for Pappworth his teaching provided an important source of income. A cup of coffee was always on offer and, despite the gruelling nature of the classes, there was, according to a number of former students, 'a great atmosphere'. Although for many young doctors the course left a hole in the pocket, they definitely felt it was worth it.

In addition (and for a considerably higher fee), some of them chose to attend Pappworth's extra tuition, in groups of four, during the late afternoon in Harley Street – doubtless keeping very quiet so as not to arouse the landlord's suspicions. A further teaching bonus Pappworth offered was the chance to attend (for a further charge, of course) weekly sessions at St John's Hospital, Battersea. In this very run-down geriatric hospital, the hand-operated lift on one occasion severed a porter's head. Here a group of paid patients served as 'long case' and 'short case' subjects.

One of his MRCP students, Dr Pat Broad (née Laird), a registrar at St John's, prepared the patients, supplying examples of different types of disease for which Pappworth would then demand a diagnosis and expatiate on symptoms and treatment. This provided a perfect opportunity to learn from one of the country's great diagnosticians, as well as a very practical preparation for the long and short cases element of the MRCP exam. Former student Professor Victor Hoffbrand also recalls attending Friern Barnet Hospital in north London to examine and talk to patients, chiefly with diseases of neurology and cardiology. This option was offered as an addition to Pappworth's normal classes. In the manner of an MRCP examiner, he would quiz groups of about a dozen students for a diagnosis.

Later in life, once Pappworth's heart condition meant that he had to reduce his teaching, he shifted operations from Seymour Hall to his home in the Vale of Health, Hampstead – after changed marital circumstances meant he had the place to himself. Classes took place once a week; as before, they lasted officially from 5pm until about 7.30pm. Pappworth was by now in his seventies, but determined to keep teaching – partly, once suspects, because he simply enjoyed having young people round to the large and lonely Queen Anne house. At the end of the evening, he would say, 'That's it. See you again.' Then he would stand by the door and collect a £10 note from everyone. (So over twenty years the cost of a Pappworth class increased tenfold.)

Dr Guy Staight, who attended these Vale of Health sessions, recalled how 'fantastic' they were. In the sitting room, twenty-five to thirty doctors would be, as in the Harley Street and Seymour Hall days, sitting on the floor. Staight was struck by how many of these doctors were Indian. They used to refer to our father as 'the guru'. I recall one of them sending him some rather dazzling Indian jewellery (to be passed on to his ladies) as a token of gratitude. A Chinese student gave him a framed, red-backgrounded set of Mandarin characters which purported to read 'Dr Pappworth – the greatest teacher in the world.' Another invited him to his wedding, and claims still to 'cherish' the crystal bowl his old teacher gave him. Whenever Helen Bamber mentioned Pappworth's name, former students would 'speak of him with nothing short of reverence'.

Those whom Pappworth taught describe his physical appearance as 'very short... a little man with a big personality... twinkly eyes, not obviously Jewish'. Very conscious of his small size (he jokingly referred to one female student, who was five foot eight inches tall, as 'towering over the dwarf'), he declared that tall people 'often have nothing in the top storey'. The giantess observed that Pappworth was 'not very smartly turned out,' and an Australian doctor who attended his classes considered that his teacher 'dressed in what we in Australia call "morning suit" – striped trousers with a black coat. This dress is only seen here on the Governor General or on Melbourne Cup Day. Because of his short size he looked slightly ludicrous and the trousers always seemed too long.' One wonders what his tailor father would have made of these sartorial judgements. According to one student, Pappworth declared that Australian students were the best: 'they're here because they want to learn, unlike you lily-livered lot.'

His students variously sum him up as 'a bit feisty... never afraid to ruffle feathers... lively, with a nice sense of humour... sprightly, very quick, quite critical, a no- nonsense and demanding teacher.' One former student, however, describes him as 'an arrogant and cynical little man, with chips on his shoulder'. Several recall that he did not suffer fools gladly. He was also considered 'quite iconoclastic'. He is remembered by some as having a slight lisp. There is no doubt that my father did pronounce certain letters with exaggerated emphasis, and 's' was one of these. Perhaps it was the pains he must have taken in earlier years to lose that trace of a Scouse accent that made his pronunciation of some words idiosyncratic. Like one of his students, I can hear his voice echo in my mind as I remember the way he said, 'eggzam', 'vairy' and 'pacific', instead of 'exam', 'very' and 'specific'.

His MRCP students felt that Pappworth took a personal interest in each of them. Helen Bamber noticed that they appeared to 'respect him immensely, even though he could also be 'very fearsome,' firing questions at great speed. Dr Barry Hoffbrand told me that, as one of his students, he could 'relate' to Pappworth 'because I admired what he was doing'. 'His sheer personality made him so memorable and his classes such an experience,' Dr Pat Broad told Allan Gaw. She revealed that Pappworth sometimes drove her from St John's Hospital to his Harley Street sessions, 'hand on my knee on one occasion'. Some years ago I was told a similar story by a female doctor whose colleague had apparently experienced this side of Dr Pappworth. These claims cast an interesting light on the man who tried to live his life according to Torah and Talmud, and speak also, perhaps, of his loneliness. He never spoke of his family, apparently.

The delivery of the MRCP classes was on a question-and-answer basis, rather than a lecture. Pappworth's teaching style was unique. It was clear and definite, his words delivered with a careful, deliberate emphasis. He would list differential signs and their causes. He would take his students through a set of diseases, asking questions and commenting on their answers, which he then used for further questioning. He encouraged them to start with the most common likely diagnosis, and to go from the general to the specific. In the case of an iron deficiency, for example, start with the haemorrhage and then move on to the question of heavy periods. He didn't just imitate a patient's strange walk: he explained it. His teaching skills might be revealed in the way he showed how a complex process, such as examination of the cranial nerves, should be carried out. He would encourage his students to look for points of difference: what causes hepatomegaly (enlarged liver) alone, what causes splenomegaly (enlarged spleen) alone, and what causes both?

A favourite phrase of Pappworth's (doubtless taken from his photographic hobby) was the 'wide-angle lens' needed to make a correct diagnosis. He advised his students to keep their eyes roving. In the exam's long and short cases, they shouldn't just examine the part they were asked to: look further, and you'll find the answer is there somewhere. Pappworth was an 'aggressive' teacher, who believed in putting his students on the spot and quizzing them individually, but this combative method 'made you think' and got 'your adrenaline running'.

According to Professor Karol Sikora, who took Pappworth's MRCP course in the early 1970s, 'Traditional medical teaching frequently involved mocking students.' Sikora himself, as a young doctor, was sworn at by his superiors in front of patients. Pappworth, however, 'was always a gent. He would never teach by mockery.' The distinction between humiliation and mockery is a narrow one, but if this can be defined it does provide a good picture of the kind of man Pappworth was – somebody always just about managing to step back from the edge of danger. He could be sharp and sarcastic if a student got something wrong. His sessions, which one student admitted she sometimes had to force herself to go to, hardened the young doctors, who often found the exam itself was mild compared to a Pappworth class. Although the intensity of his style left them feeling drained, they found that the two or more 'riveting' hours had sped by remarkably quickly.

As his students perceived it, what he wanted above all was that they should gain the confidence, for instance, to perform a physical examination properly, and to show the patient that they had this self-confidence. Thanks to Pappworth's style of teaching, his students realised that they actually knew more about medicine than they had believed. They learned not to panic, and to think logically. As one former student put it, 'I learned to keep talking some sense rather than sitting open-mouthed and silent.' 'The problem with medicine in those days,' muses Sikora, 'was that young doctors weren't given sufficient confidence or guidance.' With Pappworth, by contrast, and in spite of the aggressive style, 'you felt relaxed.'

Much of this confidence was provided by the way in which Papworth would cover a different subject each week – for example, thyroid disease one week, chest medicine the next. He would pick on one student to stand and talk on a given topic in front of the class. 'It was exacting and humiliating at times,' recalls Martin Scurr, 'but it made sure that you had read up on the subject.' Scurr adds that 'the true value was that it gave you confidence,' with the reminder that as 'slaves of the NHS' they had no teaching on the job. Pappworth was always keen to instil the confidence which emanates from having been put successfully 'on the spot', and delivered successfully.

Pappworth loved teaching. His students could tell this just by looking at his face during classes. Professor Sikora, now Dean of the Medical School at the University of Buckingham, remarked to me that Pappworth would have made a great dean of a medical school. Although there is no doubt that he relied on teaching as an important source of income, he did it mainly because he enjoyed it – and because he sensed the positive response from his students, who considered him 'a fantastic teacher'. According to Helen Bamber, 'He would impart learning... He spoke always in a rather rabbinical way,' spicing his lectures with Talmudic quotations, but he was also good at making his students laugh with him. He liked engaging with people, but tended to find that classes provided an easier forum for this than less structured social situations. He was always a great talker, but in a way that reminds me of a story told about Samuel Taylor Coleridge. The great poet and philosopher, if his interlocutor edged away, would simply carry on talking to a blank wall.

Pappworth's MRCP classes, however, offered no blank walls. They included much monologue – usually about fifteen to twenty minutes of hard facts, but broken up by what one former student describes as 'ten minutes of a virtual stand-up comedy routine (he was very funny)'. Dr Pat Broad confirms this: 'His teaching was like nothing I had before or since: it was like going to the theatre.' One former student told Allan Gaw that, even after forty years, he still consciously copied Pappworth's style of teaching, citing the 'wide angle lens' and repeating the 'you will... struggle on your own' quotation. Victor Hoffbrand was similarly influenced in his own teaching style.

Lectures were enlivened by Pappworth's vast collection of slides. These included pictures of the unusual diseases he had encountered during his career. Here his interest in photography coincided with his profession. Many of his case photographs were included in his textbook A *Primer of Medicine*, and former student Dr Guy Staight describes these as 'amazing... You'd never see anything like that anywhere else.' Lord Owen (formerly Dr David Owen, whose attendance at Pappworth's MRCP course was cut short by his election in 1966 as an MP for Plymouth) recalls 'an inspired teacher,' who offered 'little but in total important tips about diagnosis.' Advice included such nuggets as 'Get on the patient's wavelength. When it's right, you know. The diagnosis slots in'. In the exam, 'The most important thing is to start off with the main feature you're certain of and to avoid anything you're not sure of.'

He told his students to work through a physical examination zone by zone, using a methodical approach. When he took groups of students to try and diagnose cases at St John's Hospital, he wouldn't perform the physical examination himself. Instead, he watched how his students examined the patient, as though he were a mock MRCP examiner. Dr Pat Broad kept notes which included some of his favourite aphorisms. These included practical points such as 'Use good light and use a magnifying glass if necessary to look at skin lesions,' memorable epigrams like 'Think anatomy, then pathology, then specific pathology,' common-sense advice ('Give yourself three minutes at the end of the examination to collect your thoughts'), and gems such as 'When taking a history, don't waste time on the deaf or the daft.'

Apart from the MRCP courses, Pappworth continued to deliver one-off lectures: after the publication of *Human Guinea Pigs* in particular, he was much in demand. Karol Sikora vividly remembers a lecture Pappworth gave at the Hammersmith Hospital in 1970. Some young Hammersmith doctors had, against the wishes of their consultants, invited Pappworth to speak about the issues surrounding his controversial exposé. Sikora claims that there was 'no dissent from Pappworth among the younger doctors' .As we shall see in the next chapter, the Hammersmith was one of Pappworth's chief blacklist targets in *Human Guinea Pigs*. Sikora notes that its chief offending researcher, Professor Sheila Sherlock, was not present at the lecture.

Cracking the establishment's exam

So Pappworth was a 'natural teacher'. Perhaps it was in the genes; three of his sisters had become teachers, and two of his daughters followed in his pedagogic footsteps. Helen Bamber stressed in interview with Allan Gaw that he was 'very warm' with his students, 'but of course he felt he was one of them.' The students, she explained, knew that both they and Pappworth were 'up against the establishment... He was on *their* side.' Nevertheless, if he sensed that a student wasn't making the most of the opportunity given him to learn, was being inattentive or not giving of his best, he could be very stern. Bamber concedes, however, that 'he didn't impose impossibilities. He understood weakness, but he also understood strength.' He did sometimes misjudge things, nevertheless. One woman doctor remembers that, in the middle of an MRCP class, he suddenly asked her 'What is the length of a normal penis?' As her blushes deepened and her silence persisted, he joked, 'Come on – you must have some idea.' This crude sense of humour was something he seems to have remained incapable of modifying.

Why was Pappworth such an unparalleled success in getting his students through the Membership exam? One reason is feedback from candidates after the exam. Pappworth made it a condition of acceptance onto his course that candidates would feed back afterwards information about the questions they had been asked in *vivas* and 'clinicals'. He would ask them to see him after the long and short cases element of their exam, so that they could tell him about the patients they saw. This information he then passed on to future students. With the same aim, he asked them to write down, as soon as possible after they had sat the clinical exam paper, the X-rays, ECGs and pathology (for example) that they had been shown, and the precise wording of two of the written questions set, then post these details to him. He would use this information to drill his current students on why such cases might have been set, why such questions were important, and how they would have answered them.

One former attendee jokingly referred to all this as 'industrial espionage', but it is not far away from the very sensible (and expected) practice of contemporary teachers. In exams at all levels, they now simply download past papers. Not surprisingly, Pappworth could reliably predict the cases on which his students would be tested.

There appears to have been something very secretive about the Royal College of Physicians in the era when Pappworth was busy providing it with huge numbers of new Members. One former student described the relationship between the College and Pappworth as 'Gamekeeper and poacher'. Pappworth knew a great deal about the exam and, having studied their foibles, about its examiners. Some of these he mentioned by name, with advice on specific approaches to their questions should a candidate encounter one of them. He criticised and made fun of the examiners, and of some of the 'silly questions' candidates were asked. Apparently, warned Pappworth, one had a false eye, which he used to take out if you were doing really badly in your *viva*. An analytical skill Pappworth taught was how to examine, not just the patient, but the system.

A further, very simple explanation of the Pappworth courses' success is that enrollment on one entitled the student to purchase copies of the past ten or so multiple-choice papers used in the MRCP exam. Pappworth produced these himself, within days of the exam, despite the top-secret status of the paper. In many of the MRCP exam sittings, about 40 per cent of the candidates had been to Pappworth's courses – perhaps a hundred of those present. If one hundred candidates were memorising and sending him the wording of two questions, it is not surprising that Pappworth accumulated so swiftly the gold dust that would show his students what the examiners thought was important. On the more conventional topic of reading lists, Pappworth advised his students to read one of the standard medical textbooks from cover to cover, and to make marginal notes. And he warned them against wasting time by attempting to tackle books on specialist subjects.

Pappworth was a master on tips about how to pass. But he was keen that his students should not conspicuously give themselves away as Pappworth alumni when confronted by examiners. Such minor but important details were a trademark of his success. One senior doctor whom he taught described him thus: 'What Pappworth taught was like a good driving instructor. Make it clear you're looking in the rear-view mirror' during the test. Perhaps this is the kind of thing Pappworth himself had in mind when, asked once the reason for his students' high pass rate, quipped: 'I teach them tricks.'

According to one of his Australian students, he stressed from the start that he was not there to teach them medicine; his job was simply to help them pass the MRCP exam – which, in the Pappworth world-view, had nothing to do with being a good doctor. Like today's GCSEs and A Levels, it was all about jumping through hoops. Pappworth claimed that the examiners often judged a candidate by the weight of his written paper. He advised against abbreviations, and dared them to invent things if they were uncertain about the identity of, for example, some nineteenth-century doctor. Pappworth was, apparently, indignant that the College was collecting doctors' money without offering anything, apart from a diploma, in return. He clearly regarded the MRCP exam as little more than an industry, and his courses, which the elders of the profession dismissed as 'cramming', were his enterprising response.

In a letter to the *British Medical Journal* on 4 May 1963, Sir George Pickering, Regius Professor of Medicine at the University of Oxford, followed up on previous correspondence on how to improve not just the MRCP exam, but medical examinations in general. Claiming that examinations had now 'become an abuse, and what is slightly less pleasant, a vested abuse,' he declared that the best way of assessing a doctor is on performance on the job, rather than through written examination. This was the era, after all, when what we term 'continuous assessment' was becoming fashionable. He was responding to an earlier letter from Sir Robert Platt, President of the Royal College of Physicians from 1957 to 1962. Platt believed that it was possible to design genuinely effective examinations. The question of how best to test aspiring and recently qualified doctors was one which Pappworth was not alone in raising.

From the 1950s to the 1980s, when Pappworth was teaching, the MRCP exam was far more clinical than it is now. Especially important, therefore, was his teaching of clinical skills. These, according to one former student, were generally during that era 'really badly taught'. Pappworth delighted in these skills, which were to him 'a fine art'. He insisted that it was the patient who often gave you the vital clues. If the doctor listened to him, observing him carefully, it should be possible to reach a diagnosis. 'His observation of the patient was paramount and very important,' is one of the chief lessons absorbed by Helen Bamber.

An Australian student recalls a Pappworth lecture entitled 'The Hand'. Assume the examiner has asked you to examine a patient's hand and consider what you are looking for. Pappworth started with what you might notice about the nails, then the joints, skin, pigmentation, sweating or lack of it, and tremor. Similar lectures on the chest and heart were also memorable features of the course. The detailed, systematic method by which Pappworth taught his students to use that 'wide-angle lens' in examining and assessing patients, and to put together different signs in order to reach a diagnosis, offered a path to exam success paved with excellent clinical practice. Exam strategies, as Pappworth was fiercely aware, were a necessary follow-up to good clinical skills. One sub-radar technique suggested by Pappworth for candidates in the long case test was simply to find out how much the patient himself knew. Tell him, urged Pappworth *sotto voce*, you think he is suffering from 'A' and then ask him if that is what the doctors have told him; tell him that you would do 'B' tests and ask him if he has had others; ask if there are any X-rays to hand and then look at them.

Pappworth's students carried away with them, not just the coveted Membership, but also a deep-seated respect for the sick person, and a sense also that here in their teacher was someone who respected them. He was keenly aware of the important stage they had reached in their career, and of the need to give them courage as they feared being shrugged aside by those who had done the same to him. He understood their apprehensiveness as they went into the exam, and their dread of being humiliated. One of the reasons his students were so grateful to Pappworth was that they always knew he was on their side.

The reason Pappworth himself gives for his courses' success is that 'it was considered by the medical establishment that there were too many registrars trying to climb the slippery ladder to consultant, and their remedy was to reduce the pass rates for all postgraduate medical diplomas'. At one point during the 1950s, the MRCP pass rate dropped below five per cent. This was the figure when Professor David London, one of Pappworth's early students and later Registrar of the Royal College of Physicians, first attempted the exam. By the time he succeeded at the second attempt, the pass rate had risen to ten per cent.

The whole system seems to have been very arbitrary. At every exam, however – and exams were held four times a year – Pappworth's students formed never less than thirty-three percent, and usually about fifty per cent, of the successful candidates. On one occasion, only twenty-eight young doctors passed the MRCP. Of these, twenty-two were Pappworth's students. 'The notion rapidly developed that it was very difficult to pass that exam without attending my classes.' Doubtless part of the appeal of running the course was, for Pappworth, a chance to strike out alone on an enterprise unconnected with the medical establishment, and one which had the power to draw attention to what he saw as deficiencies in medical education at the time.

Pappworth was, above all, a diagnostician who happened also to be a brilliant teacher on holistic clinical questions: how to approach, examine, talk to and assess a patient. His students valued his teaching, not just because it manoeuvred them through the MRCP exam, but also because it helped them learn how to analyse symptoms and signs, and ask the appropriate questions in developing a diagnosis. Pappworth knew how to talk to his patients, to make them feel comfortable, and monitor that he wasn't causing distress. His students learned how to follow this vital formula: he showed them, in the words of Karol Sikora, how to 'be kind to the patient; don't embarrass them; remove only the amount of clothing that needs to be removed for an examination; make sure all clothing is given back discreetly.'

According to Guy Staight, Pappworth had a 'great manner' with his patients, whom 'he loved'. He constantly stressed the importance of the doctor's relationship with the patient: after all, if you allow him to tell you the story, 'you're there'. A patient's tale will, in the end, reveal the diagnosis. The skills of critical analysis required of the physician – the ability to weigh risks against benefits – were forcefully communicated by Pappworth to his students, one of whom described this emphasis as 'very Pappworth'. As physician and teacher, Pappworth was greatly interested in the whole process of making clinical decisions and in showing younger doctors how to plot a patient's course. He taught them how to think in terms of regions of the body, and how to distinguish between signs common to several conditions.

A mixture of tests and judgement are always required. Into this formula Pappworth diffused the 'one human' approach, rather than damming off all possible areas in favour of single-stream specialisation. Pappworth stressed how important it is to be able to make a judgement early on: how urgent is this case? He was adept at putting together the clinical signs along with the history and then making decisions about the next step. It is not surprising that Staight, like other former students, continued to contact Pappworth for professional advice, telephoning him when they had diagnostic puzzles. As a mentor as much as a teacher, Pappworth, people knew, could always be relied on. It may have been difficulties in his personal life which made him all the more ready to give up his time to help people he liked – especially those in his profession.

Like all great physicians, Pappworth – and those whom he taught – knew instinctively that to get the diagnosis, at the bedside, is a matter of pride for the doctor. Tests merely confirm what a good physician can work out. For Pappworth, one of the great dangers he saw gathering in his lifetime was that the impressive battery of tests becoming widely available might take the doctor's foot off the controls and render him clinically lazy. But there was no chance that those taught by Pappworth would be tempted to rely wholly on exciting new technology. One important achievement of his MRCP classes was to boost doctors' morale, convincing each of them that they would never be replaced by machines, and that they, when they replaced those currently leading the medical profession, had it in them to be just as good if not better than their predecessors.

'I have no doubts,' declared one former student, 'I would never have passed the exam without Pappworth. I felt the money was well spent and did not begrudge it.' Another, in considering Pappworth's influence in making doctors think carefully about how they were treating their patients as human beings, described him as 'a sort of John the Baptist'.

One benefit of passing the exam was the invitation issued to all new Members to a celebratory dinner at the Royal College of Physicians, which Fellows also attended. Tradition has it that Pappworth would always arrive late, at which point his successful candidates would rise to their feet and applaud him as he walked to his seat. This was interpreted as a firecracker launched at Fellows hostile to their guru.

Pappworth records in his memoir that on the four evenings a week that he held his classes, 'I never got home till after 8pm. I am certain that neither Jean nor any of my daughters ever appreciated, and still do not appreciate, how hard I worked.' I personally can remember only that Wednesday was the one night of the week when we knew our father would be home late because he was teaching. This must have been after he had dropped his classes from four to one evening a week. So it was on a Wednesday that our mother allowed us the thrill of creating our own shish-kebabs for dinner – the practice of dipping our metal skewers into a pan of frying oil being, doubtless, something of which she knew her husband would disapprove.

Our father muses in his recorded memoir that 'Workaholics rarely get the appreciation from those who positively but indirectly benefit from their labours, which makes me cynically ask myself, was it all worthwhile?' He then consoles himself with the reminder that, over the years, he coached over 1600 candidates for the Membership exam. These comprised a very sizeable percentage of those who passed, and passed at the first attempt.

Pappworth continued to rent his consulting room at number 66, and remained proud of his Harley Street address. Although he benefited by practising from such an élite location, it did represent for him the entrenched nature of British medicine's idiosyncrasies.

Another source of income for Pappworth during our childhood was the work he did for life assurance companies: his task was to assess those cases about which there were doubts as to physical fitness, or the insurance demanded. The only time I recall him mentioning this at home was when, contrary to protocol, he gave us the name of a well-known comedian he had examined. Another, more surprising, branch-line he travelled was as a ringside doctor at boxing matches – a sport through which some Jewish immigrants found they could integrate. Years later, his son-in-law Saul Waranch, a keen amateur boxer in his native Dallas, tried asking Maurice about his experiences at the ringside, but found his father-in-law reticent on the subject. Saul recalled that 'he lambasted boxing, saying that it was not really a sport, there were too many head injuries and it should be banned.'

Pappworth was certainly never short of patients. Doctors – many taught by him – would send difficult cases his way. They would send him members of their family who were ill – the greatest compliment one doctor can pay another. Through their contacts overseas, they sent him patients from abroad. Little surprise that he became known as 'the doctors' doctor'. Helen Bamber points out that even after the medical establishment had closed ranks on Pappworth – long before the publication of *Human Guinea Pigs* – the steady flow of patients to 66 Harley Street never abated. In Bamber's words, though 'he was ostracised, [and] yes they clobbered him and they didn't allow him a consultancy and they kept him out,' his reputation as a great physician meant that he remained the doctor of choice. If the diagnosis looked complicated, Pappworth was your man.

Bamber recalls in her interview with Allan Gaw how, when her husband was seriously ill with viral pneumonia, and appeared to be dying, she brought Pappworth to the hospital to take a look at him. She describes the scene as 'one of the most moving things of my life'. Many of the young doctors at the hospital, hearing that Pappworth was on his way to see a patient, all gathered round the bed 'where Pappworth was proclaiming, as he did – you know, hands going, moving around and so on – and I think he saved his life.'

'A Primer of Medicine': clarity and charity

Of those students who prepared for their MRCP through faithful attendance at Pappworth's courses, many backed this up with close study of his textbook, *A Primer of Medicine*. 'Every night I read the *Primer*,' recalls one. 'There was a bit of philosophy in there we all laughed at, but it was the best medical textbook.' Others were less enthusiastic, one doctor even telling me that the first edition was full of mistakes. Helen Bamber herself maintained that the *Primer* was, in her opinion, better written than *Human Guinea Pigs*. But nothing came close to the experience of being taught by him in person.

A Primer of Medicine was first published in 1960. The publisher, Butterworths, brought out four further editions, the fifth and last appearing in 1984. Pappworth was insistent that, this being such a personal work and no ordinary textbook, he did not want any subsequent editions written by others. After his death, the family was placed in a difficult position, with an old American medical friend of his, Dr Dennis Bloomfield, and also a well-qualified young British doctor asking us to entrust them with the honour of a sixth edition. It was a hard decision, but we eventually felt that we had to follow our father's wishes – in the full knowledge, of course, that the Pappworth *Primer* would all too soon become out of date and therefore unread.

Part of what makes the *Primer* so idiosyncratic is its root in Pappworth's Judaism, and indeed in the ethics of all great religions and philosophies. Its preface includes, among other quotations, the words of Nachmanides, also known as Ramban (acronym for Rabbi Moses ben Nachman), a physician, philosopher, mystic and poet, who lived in Catalonia until the Spanish Inquisition forced him to flee to the Holy Land in 1267: 'I do not consider myself a donkey carrying books... I will plead in all modesty, but will judge according to the sight of my own eyes.' That is indeed characteristic of Pappworth's attitudes, and one which he wished to convey to his students: carefully examine the evidence before you.

In his first chapter he examines the ethical precepts as propounded by great thinkers, and also considers ethical codes. Those whose words he cites range from Plato to the judge and legal thinker Lord Denning, quoting from the latter's Earl Grey Memorial lecture of 1953: 'Without religion there can be no morality and without morality there can be no law.' The key to Pappworth's human morality lies in 'the Golden Rule', and he cites the various sources of its most important principle. 'Love they neighbour as thyself,' the Book of Leviticus commands us. In the first century BC, Rabbi Hillel advised 'What is hateful to you, never do to your fellow men.' Matthew in his Gospel makes the same point slightly differently: 'Whatsoever you would that men should do to you, do you even so to them.' Pappworth blames the 'unhealthy and livid condition of modern society' on 'ever-diminishing spirituality contrasted with an ever-increasing domination by the intellectual vulgarity of the mass media'. There must have been students who, confronted by this stark opening to what they expected to be a medical textbook, were not only very surprised but, possibly, rather alienated.

Pappworth expresses his regret that it is no longer customary for graduating doctors to take the Hippocratic Oath, much of which is 'still sound', despite its 'obsolete' elements. He explains his reasoning: 'Today..., when medicine is rapidly becoming dehumanized because of emphasis on laboratory procedures and the domination of many medical schools by research workers, it is becoming more and more necessary that all doctors prescribe to, and earnestly and meticulously follow, an agreed ethical code.'

Pappworth was ready with his own suggested new code, which would include an awareness of the doctor's responsibilities to both the medical profession and to the community. '[T]he health and welfare of my patients will always be my prime consideration and not what may be deemed for the good of society or the advancement of science and medical knowledge... I will never knowingly harm a patient or do anything which I would not readily agree to being done in similar circumstances to myself or a close relative... I will never submit my patient to any surgical operation or investigation without the patient's valid consent.'

Chapter Two, which opens with an epigraph from Corinthians, is entitled 'Learning and Teaching Clinical Medicine'. Pappworth expresses his shock at the inability of some medical students to diagnose commonly occurring conditions, and espouses the learning of facts. This is not in a Gradgrind sense of the word, but springs from Pappworth's emphasis on the simple truth that we need to know things in order to be able to act. 'It is impossible to be a good clinician without knowing many facts,' when it comes to making a diagnosis or prescribing a drug. 'Factual knowledge is not acquired by inspiration, but only by techniques of memorizing and hard work.' He laments that the study of anatomy has been downgraded in so many medical schools, teaching being now more focused on biochemistry and electro-physics. Once again, the car-driving analogy becomes useful: it is possible to drive a car more than competently, argues Pappworth, with no knowledge at all of the laws of thermodynamics or the internal combustion engine. A good motor mechanic will recognise the cause of an abnormal noise in a car even if he has no knowledge of physics. The analogy shows Pappworth the clinician as a man who placed the practical skills gained from knowledge and experience above academic theory. The important point, however, was that it is possible to become a good doctor through hard work and the intelligent application of those unfashionable 'facts'. The art of teaching, on the other hand, he claimed to be 'a special skill, and few have a natural gift for it'.

Pappworth himself had the gift of imparting information while at the same time making classes not just interesting but positively enjoyable. 'The most important pedagogic method is teaching by example. Furthermore, a teacher must never be afraid of admitting ignorance and be prepared to follow the dictum

104

that ignorance about a subject is an excellent reason for preserving silence.' This last Pappworthism certainly had a big influence on my life, and on the life of my youngest sister: sitting round the dining room table at home, we were too terrified to leap in with our own opinions. We were much too worried about being wrong. It was only after we had left home that we realised we actually knew rather a lot, and our views were worth expressing. Pappworth was perhaps less successful in instilling self-confidence in two of his daughters than in his students. Our middle sister, Dinah, was never afraid to fight back, and life in the Pappworth family as we grew up was frequently enlivened by arguments between a father and daughter who believed their opinion was always worth airing.

Many of Pappworth's educational aphorisms in the *Primer* are wise, and testament to the reading and thinking he did about teaching in general and the teaching of medicine in particular. Had he been given the opportunity, he might have transformed medical education in the UK. In a way, he did – from the side-lines. He pleads for a 'return to the famous tradition of clinical teaching which was formerly the pride of British medicine, a tradition which insisted that it must begin and continue at the bedside, using books, lectures and audio-visual aids as mere supplements'. For Pappworth, no epitaph could pay better tribute than that selected by Sir William Osler: 'He taught medicine in the wards.' Speaking to medical teachers, Pappworth advises them to 'guide their pupils without pampering them, and to help them without being meddlesome. The teacher must exhibit a vibrant enthusiasm, and give something of himself so that, in the words of Samuel Johnson, "New things are made familiar and familiar things made new."'

Naturally, Pappworth's pet bugbears appear as he expounds his theories on medical education. The blame for poor teaching lies with the rush to research. 'Research is an essential university activity, but unfortunately many teaching hospitals have become primarily research institutions where teaching and the care of patients are secondary.' This criticism sadly applies now, as we reach the half-centenary of *Human Guinea Pigs*: many undergraduates in many disciplines complain about the quality of the teaching, and the lack of contact time.

Pappworth's analysis still rings true. Academic promotion comes not from great teaching, but from research (described as exhaling a 'halo of glamour') and the number of publications produced. Every physician, on the other hand, 'should proudly recognize that his bedside techniques and use of laboratory findings can transform him into a true scientist'. Pappworth also laments the tendency to over-specialise: 'After such long exposure to the outpourings of super-specialists and researchers, it is a miracle that any young graduates wish to become general practitioners, and the lost enthusiasm for general practice is wholly deplorable.'

Although the reader can become irritated by the numerous quotations, from Alexander Pope to George Bernard Shaw, there is also plenty to arouse a wry smile. Most of us will recognise the truth behind Pappworth's claim that teachers who supply their students with long reading lists use this as an excuse for not actually teaching them. 'Fortunately,' he adds, 'most students ignore them.' He also writes about ward rounds and outpatient clinics, and why students should be taught to present cases: 'Few medicals, whatever their status, seem capable of presenting cases in a satisfactory manner at clinical meetings, conferences, ward rounds or at examinations. Too often they are unmitigated bores.' No wonder so many in the medical profession disliked Maurice Pappworth.

Pappworth attached great importance to clear and accurate language, and was suspicious of all verbal ambiguity. The third chapter of the *Primer* is devoted to 'Medical Vocabulary'. Typically turning this into something of a joke, he criticises 'the fashionable habit of quibbling about the meanings of such commonly used words as "bronchitis", "emphysema" and "dyspnoea", which leads to long-winded discussions concerning short-winded patients.' Reading his pronouncement that 'Words can be used to confuse, to cloak ignorance, to mislead,' it is worth bearing in mind that the first edition of the Primer came out only eleven years after Orwell's *Nineteen Eighty-Four*. Pappworth, an educator wary of neologisms, is scornful of the word 'testees' for candidates sitting multiple choice papers. A particularly conspicuous red rag was the rather meaningless word 'parameter', whose use has spread with vengeful rapidity since Pappworth's day. I can vividly recall his excitement when, consulting the Oxford English Dictionary, he discovered that the word 'jargon' derives (as encountered in Romantic poetry) from 'A noise like the twittering of birds' – a nugget of information he includes in this chapter.

Pappworth had a lively and colourful written style, which may go some way to explaining his impatience with those who had to fall back on jargon, 'gibberish, gobbledegook, codswallop and mental garbage'. He was also full of wisdom when it came to explaining why words matter, and I remember him giving me the advice that he offers here to readers: 'There is no such thing as either a "never" or an "always" in clinical medicine; "never" means "hardly

106

ever" and "always" means "nearly always."' Not surprisingly, Pappworth remained suspicious of statistics, which he compares to bikinis, 'concealing what is vital and revealing much that is occasionally interesting'.

Chapter Four brings us to 'The Art and Science of Diagnosis'. Pappworth describes diagnosis as a 'creative art', which 'belongs to the realm of discovery. It is detective work controlled by a system of logical analysis... Medicine is both an art and a science.' Diagnosis, he insists, should be based on a triplet of 'history, physical signs and investigations'. In the twenty-first century it is the battery of technically sophisticated 'investigations' which dominates diagnosis and the follow-up of a disease's progress. The Pappworth rule book may appear somewhat outdated. But most patients would, I believe, like to see modern machines combined with the time, sympathy and expertise of a knowledgeable physician. This was how my own unusual disease was diagnosed.

Indeed, Pappworth was convinced that the growing emphasis on technological developments was keeping doctors away from patients: 'A grain of clinical judgement is worth a ton of biochemical results.' I found, in conversation with some leading contemporary doctors, that many in the profession are now alarmed, thirty-six years on from the fifth edition of the *Primer*, by the knee-jerk tendency to order far more tests and investigations than are actually needed – 'like an uncritical shopper in a supermarket', as Pappworth expresses it. As with his concerns about unnecessary clinical research, he was acutely aware that some of these superfluous investigations might well bring 'discomfort... and possible hazards' to the patient.

'History Taking' is the fifth chapter, and here the student reader will find much of the common sense – and the ability to convey this – for which Pappworth was renowned. So often it is the simple things which can make the most difference, if they are remembered. The doctor who has absorbed Pappworth's advice that 'A correct diagnosis is often missed, not because of lack of knowledge but because of not listening attentively to the patient or not asking the appropriate question' is likely to become a very good physician. History taking should, Pappworth suggests, 'be evolved like a well-written narrative with a literary form and style. Patients will usually answer all questions properly if properly presented at the proper time.'

The alliteration here is almost certainly deliberate – part of Pappworth's pedagogic technique, with its memorably aphoristic style. As in his lectures to his MRCP students, Pappworth emphasises the importance of using one's eyes, closely observing the patient from the moment he walks into the room. Much of this advice he was to repeat in his final book, *Passing Medical Examinations*, in which he gave valuable tips on how to diagnose 'the long case'. Pappworth, described by James Le Fanu as 'the standard-bearer of the tradition of clinical methods,' emphasised throughout the Primer the superiority, when making a diagnosis, of history taking and examination over the tests and investigations 'vigorously promoted by the clinical scientists'.

The culmination of this chapter occurs when Pappworth alights on one of his most treasured topics – the doctor-patient relationship. 'A good doctor patient relationship,' he declares, 'depends on mutual trust and respect... We must attempt to make the patient appreciate that we recognize him as an individual... It is only by adopting a friendly, warm, gracious and good-mannered attitude that we will obtain the confidence of many patients, and complete confidence is essential for good histories. Arousing in a patient the belief that you are concerned whole-heartedly with his welfare greatly assists, or even may produce, therapeutic benefits.'

An old school-friend of mine, normally terrified of the eccentric Dr Pappworth, told me about the occasion when he visited her in a psychiatric nursing home: she was recovering from a nervous breakdown. My father at that moment became a completely different person from the one she had previously encountered. He was kind, empathetic, gentle. He sat by the bed and listened to her. Another friend was referred to him by his mother, a fellow doctor. My father visited him at home, and apparently the moment he walked into the room it was clear that he understood the problem. Again, he was a model of what he himself called 'the physician-friend'.

This was not a side of Maurice Pappworth encountered by many of those who didn't happen to be his patients. One particular female patient, with a tremulous, sad little voice, would telephone our home from time to time and ask to speak to our father. To his three daughters this became a source of some hilarity. But he always got up and went into the privacy of the coat cupboard where the telephone lived, and spent time just listening to her. Here, clearly, was not a mistress but a woman in need of kindness. I suspect our mother felt that this kindness might have been expended more liberally on her as well.

'There is usually a way of telling the truth without removing all hope': Pappworth always tried to help undergraduates and young doctors understand what it must be like to be a patient, or the close relative of someone gravely ill. He comes out with unexpected but arguably valid statements such as, when considering the physical examination, 'Uncovering the body often makes uncovering of the mind much easier.' Like the psychoanalysts of whom he was so suspicious, Pappworth recognises that more spontaneous talk may come from the couch, rather than the chair. At the end of the consultation, the Pappworth formula is for the physician to ask the patient to repeat what he has been told, so that any misunderstandings can be immediately put right.

Alongside the case studies, the photographs of diseases to be deciphered and the practical guidance, Pappworth's *Primer of Medicine* teaches its readers much about people, about society and about life. That is what makes it such an unusual and unparalleled textbook. In the Royal College of Physicians' Munks Roll, Stephen Lock's verdict on the *Primer* is that 'it was not a comprehensive account even of elementary medicine and it reads in a curiously leaden way compared with the incisiveness of his spoken talks.' But then Pappworth wasn't trying to be comprehensive, and it would have been very hard to match in a textbook the legendary impact of his classes and lectures.

Drawing on his mine of rabbinic quotations, Pappworth used to claim that he learned more from his students than from anyone else. What, in practical terms, did he gain from teaching those many hundreds of MRCP candidates? One outcome – possibly the most critically significant of his career – was that Pappworth, standing outside the magic circle of the medical establishment, picked up from his students what was going on. Then he embarked on a comprehensive reading programme, scouring the medical journals. And so *Human Guinea Pigs* was born.

Chapter Five

Breaking the silence: a rebel and his cause

'Clinical research must go on but there must be acknowledged and observed safeguards for the patients. At present such safeguards are virtually non-existent.'

(Maurice Pappworth, article in the British Medical Journal, 1963)

The secret shame of hospital research

Concerns about human experimentation, shared by other doctors, dated back to the early 1950s. Alex Paton, a registrar at the Hammersmith Hospital, wrote a private diary about the research into liver disease in which he was participating. The Hammersmith, which at the time of Pappworth's preparation of *Human Guinea Pigs* during the 1950s and 1960s housed the British Postgraduate Medical School, was one of the chief targets of his book. Indeed, of all the British hospitals mentioned in his 'blacklist', the Hammersmith appears most frequently.

One reason the Hammersmith was primarily a research hospital was that its doctors were not permitted to engage in private practice. They were essentially academic scientists. And there, at their fingertips, were patients who, during the 1950s and 1960s, often stayed in hospital for as long as six weeks if they were undergoing a procedure. Researchers would scour the wards for potential subjects. There was even a prisoner from Wormwood Scrubs who used to visit the Hammersmith for treatment and to take part in experiments. No doubt for him this offered a welcome escape from incarceration, whatever the risks. Situated in a (then) working-class area of London, the Hammersmith treated patients who tended to be in awe of their doctors. They lacked the social and educational confidence to question the necessity of procedures such as liver biopsies – which they were dishonestly assured would do them good. Not surprisingly, at no British hospital were experiments performed on private patients.

The British Postgraduate Medical School at the Hammersmith, at this time under the direction of Sir John McMichael and Dr Edward Sharpey-Schafer, became the UK's leading institution for medical research. With regard to un-ethical experimentation, the Hammersmith was then, in the words of Professor Karol Sikora, 'the worst offender'. The hospital pioneered cardiac catheterisa-tion, which, as we have seen in the Introduction, Pappworth found particularly unsavoury. According to Alex Paton's diary, at the Hammersmith there was no such thing as a consent form. This was later confirmed to me by a doctor who worked there during the 1960s. It was, wrote Paton, a case of 'yes doctor, of course doctor'.

Although Paton insisted that most of his colleagues were 'intelligent re-searchers... trying to establish new treatments and procedures that would ben-efit humanity as a whole,' he noticed that 'many of them did take liberties with patients'. In his 1964 obituary of Sir John McMichael in the *British Medical Journal*, even his close colleague Sharpey-Schafter admitted that the director of the British Postgraduate Medical School 'could seem casual in his approach to patients'. Similarly, the *BMJ*'s 2002 obituary of Pappworth's chief *bête noire*, Professor Sheila Sherlock, conceded that 'there was little place for good taste or patients' feelings'.

In a diary entry dated 17 December 1952, Paton writes: 'We and anyone else at Hammersmith use subjects for experiments who will not necessarily benefit by them. In all cases we explain what we are going to do, and the choice of whether he should submit is left to the patient. But it is of course obviously impossible to convey to the patient exactly what is meant by a hepatic catheter-isation for example... Our own experiments are usually quite harmless, but they involve quite a lot of discomfort to the patient, and the obvious question one should ask oneself is: would I submit myself to catheterisation?... The danger in a hospital such as Hammersmith is that one comes to regard patients as suit-able or otherwise for the particular procedure that one is interested in carrying out... The beds are really nothing more than an annexe to the medical labora-tories.' Paton's attitude is a striking example of someone disturbed by what he was doing but confining his concerns to the privacy of a diary, rather than choosing to blow the whistle.

Paton also considered, in a diary entry dated 27 July 1952, the case at an American hospital flagged up by Professor Henry Beecher of the Harvard Med-ical School, in which orphaned children were chosen for an experiment to study infective hepatitis. 'There is course quite a risk that a few of these children would subsequently develop cirrhosis, and considering that they already have the burden of being orphans to bear, such a thing seems quite unjustified and even criminal. There is not really very much difference between this and the methods of the Nazis.' Not only is Paton drawing a parallel between Nazi medical atrocities and the practices of contemporary American doctors which Pappworth was to echo; he is also anticipating what the author of *Human Guinea Pigs* drew attention to – namely, that it was all too often the most vulnerable members of society who were selected as experimental subjects.

Lord (Robert) Winston, later a pioneer of IVF treatment, was a researcher at the Hammersmith Hospital. In *Bad Ideas: An Arresting History of our Inventions* (2010), he recalled his colleagues' furious condemnation of Pappworth's revelations about research carried out there during the 1950s and 1960s. Winston describes such figures as those who 'loathe criticism'. Like Paton, he did not however air any concerns he may have had about unethical research.

On 14 May 1955, Dr S. Sevitt wrote to *The Lancet* expressing concerns about research carried out at the Hammersmith by Professor Sherlock. Later a Dame, she was one of the most famous doctors of her time. When the new Royal Free Hospital was built in Hampstead in 1974, she practised her research into liver disease across the entire tenth floor. Nearly twenty years before, Sevitt worried that the way in which new information was being obtained 'raises moral and ethical questions... Were the patients consulted before substances potentially dangerous to them were given and did they agree to participate in the experiments?... Medical research workers who are concerned with human lives have to steer carefully between the production of fruitful work and the obligations of the Hippocratic oath.'

This letter was music to Pappworth's ears, focusing as it did on the issue of genuinely informed consent, and the doctor's ethical obligations to his patient. He wrote immediately to *The Lancet* congratulating Sevitt on 'having the courage to write and you, for publishing a brilliant letter asking Dr Sherlock some very pertinent questions'. Describing the distinction drawn by Sherlock between an experiment and a 'therapeutic trial' as 'a piece of casuistic sophistry', he took the opportunity to launch a personal attack. For over twelve years, he claimed, Sherlock 'has been doing such and contributing many equally odious accounts to the medical literature'.

He referred to her 'dastardly experiments', declared that British teaching hospitals were 'dominated by ghoulish physiologists masquerading as clinicians', and called for their place to be 'taken by true physicians whose main interest is the welfare of their patients and not the publication of papers'. The colourful vocabulary anticipates some of the language, condemned by his critics as much too emotive, Pappworth was to use in *Human Guinea Pigs*. Not surprisingly, despite sharing many of Pappworth's views, editor Theodore Fox declined to publish his letter. 'We cannot accept it in its present form', he explained. Fox continued: 'I know that there are times when good comes of speaking strongly and by giving maximum publicity to what appear to be public scandals; but you haven't yet persuaded us here that this is one of those occasions.'

Pappworth fought back, prophesying in a letter to Fox a few days later: 'My fear is that the day may not be far distant when the whole problem will come into the public eye with the maximum publicity and the production of a grave public scandal with consequent serious damage to public confidence in the hospital service and the medical profession.' It was Pappworth himself who was to bring the problem 'into the public eye with the maximum publicity'.

Pappworth experienced difficulty in getting his letters published in medical journals. Although the *World Medical Journal* conceded in 1955 that 'There are undoubtedly some who have failed to resist an inclination for morbid curiosity', and a 1962 editorial in the *BMJ* admitted that 'probably too many pointless investigations have been made', the establishment ranks were starting to close. Pappworth received an interesting letter dated 25 May 1964 from Donald Acheson, later to become Chief Medical Officer of the UK: he had evidently been put under pressure to withdraw a letter to the *BMJ* supportive of Pappworth. When Pappworth tried the national press, he did not necessarily meet with any more success. The assistant editor of *The Observer*, for example, had cause in August 1964 to explain to Pappworth why his 'rather long letter' couldn't be published. Pappworth was an extraordinarily dogged and courageous campaigner, but one can begin to understand why editors might have found this something of a trial.

Although he was aware of fellow doctors on both sides of the Atlantic who shared his views, Pappworth continued to be disappointed by the slow rate of progress in implementing guidelines on medical ethical practice at both a national and international level. He remained pessimistic about the Nuremberg Code's chances of gaining respect. As he was to explain later in *Human Guinea Pigs*, 'the judgement rendered by the Nuremberg Military Tribunal concerning human experimentation has never been and probably never will be construed either in Britain or America as legal precedent'. In 1954, a number of research units in Britain had rejected the Medical Research Council's suggestion that patients taking part in experiments should always be asked for written consent, on the somewhat irrational grounds that such a formality would undermine patients' trust in their doctors. Ten years later, the 1964 Declaration of Helsinki, effectively the successor to the Nuremberg Code, remained precisely that: a declaration rather than an edict with enforceable powers. It had been developed for the World Medical Association by Hugh Clegg, editor of the *British Medical Journal* from 1947 to 1965. As far as Pappworth was concerned, the Declaration achieved little more than the Nuremberg Code which, similarly, was not a binding document under international law. It is important here to keep in mind the distinction between laws and regulations – that for which one might be liable for criminal prosecution, and that which is essentially a flouting of professional guidelines.

In an anonymous article published in the *BMJ* in July 1963, Pappworth argued the case for a seriously-intentioned code. 'No-one who conducts experiments on human beings can really free himself from all bias in forming an ethical judgement of what he does. That is why he needs guidelines in the shape of a code.' It was not that Pappworth was categorically against medical experimentation per se – something which his adversaries chose to misinterpret. 'Clinical research must go on,' he wrote in the *BMJ*, 'but there must be acknowledged and observed safeguards for the patients. At present such safeguards are virtually non-existent.' A few years later he was complaining that 'today we have proliferated scientific devices to keep doctors away from patients'. If they weren't experimenting on them, apparently, they were ignoring them, too busy playing with their new high-tech toys. Pappworth recognised that the best way of drawing attention to the wrongs being done to British hospital patients was to galvanise the attention of the public, and to create national headlines. There's still little the media love more than a scandalous medical story. So he continued to gather his evidence.

Interestingly, at the time Pappworth started to peel off the layers hiding unethical experiments during the 1950s, there was considerably more regulation protecting animal subjects than their human counterparts. In *Human Guinea Pigs*, Pappworth was able to observe that 'Human experiments are less trouble and... at present no form-filling or record-keeping is necessary before a human experiment is undertaken; with animals both are necessary.' Nearly always, by law, the animal had to be anaesthetised beforehand; in the case of many experiments on a man, woman or child – not necessarily. An experimenter would obviously prefer the 'subject' to be conscious, for the possible side-effects of an anaesthetic not to be an issue.

'In England', Pappworth claimed towards the end of *Human Guinea Pigs*, 'there appears to be more concern for the welfare of animals than for that of sick patients.' He pointed out that, unlike human experimentation, that on animals was strictly controlled by Act of Parliament. Before an animal experiment was undertaken, a licence was needed, and to obtain this the experimenters had to 'state in detail the purpose and nature of what they were proposing to do'. He contrasts this with the attitude to human experimentation which, for Iain Macleod (health minister between 1952 and 1955), 'is essentially one of medical ethics' and therefore requiring no law. Pointing out these skewed priorities, Pappworth returns to Nuremberg territory: 'Hitler when he first assumed power issued an edict making all animal experiments illegal. But this he followed up by ordering the mass murder of inmates of mental hospitals.'

The British public's traditional concern for animal welfare was eventually matched by growing demands for the rights of men and woman at a time when huge developments in medical technology were matched by the decline of deference.

Now he and Helen Bamber, his colleague from St George's, Wapping, began to compile their case archive. One particularly striking fact which they uncovered was that, in Britain at least, risky experimentations were never carried out on private patients. They reserved such procedures, Pappworth drily observed near the beginning of *Human Guinea Pigs*, 'for what is known as the "hospital class"'. He emphasised that one was very unlikely, in the UK, to become the subject of experimentation if admitted to a non-teaching hospital for routine treatment. 'But if the hospital were a teaching or associated one, that remote chance becomes a distinct possibility although not a probability.'

According to Bamber, it was 'the lack of real communication with the person about what and why the intervention would take place' that 'upset' Pappworth, and made him 'very uneasy'. It was in large part the 'first-hand reports' of his postgraduate students that, according to *Human Guinea Pigs*, confirmed 'what I have seen myself. Adequate, let alone full, explanations are often not given to patients. Possible complications and real dangers are hardly ever hinted at.'

Doctors would ask their junior staff to find a certain number of control patients. The experimenters themselves frequently had no direct contact with the patients themselves prior to the procedure. House physicians 'do not know why... a certain patient is missing from his ward on a certain day'. These were some of the stories Pappworth heard from his students. He also scoured as many as possible of the reports on experiments published in the 162 British medical journals and six thousand such journals produced worldwide. There was plenty to be found, given that the path to career promotion, then as now – especially in academic circles – was through the publication of research. In *The Rise and Fall of British Medicine*, James Le Fanu describes this as 'the sort of degenerate "scientism"' that ran completely counter to the work of the great clinicians and diagnosticians'.

The first salvo: 'Human Guinea Pigs: A Warning'

Pappworth's first important break came in 1962 when he was asked to contribute an article to the literary quarterly magazine *Twentieth Century*. Its autumn edition was given over to the subject of 'Doctors in the Sixties'. Allan Gaw describes the article as 'an early salvo in the battle against unethical research practices', and its strapline promises a 'disturbing report'. Citing mostly examples from British hospitals, but also including four American cases, Pappworth aimed to convey to the layman the abuses taking place. *Twentieth Century* was not a medical magazine: it was aimed at the intelligent general reader. This prepared the ground for Pappworth's style in *Human Guinea Pigs*, whose target audience was likewise lay members of the public interested in matters medical, moral, legal and ethical.

Pappworth's written style may have avoided medical jargon, but it certainly pulled no punches in employing controversially strong rhetoric. His opening sentence claimed that 'During the last twenty years clinical medicine in British teaching hospitals has become dominated by research workers who are primarily experimentalists, rarely having any interest in patients purely as patients.' He drew attention to the fact that 'each individual procedure carries with it a risk of killing the patient,' which 'has never been denied'. He showed himself to be characteristically sceptical of sweeping claims: 'the commonly reiterated phrase, "it was done for the good of society" has a Marxian and Hitlerian ring, and is unacceptable.'

Critically, as always, he focused on the question of informed consent: 'the real crux of the matter is this. Did all the patients really give full consent, after honest and detailed explanation of what was to be meted out to them?' As he was to do in his book five years later, Pappworth described in squirm-inducing detail what was done to patients during some of these experiments. And the full force of his criticism fell on those who, from curiosity rather than necessity,

116

experimented on children – the least 'defensible, legally and morally' of all his examples. 'Parents may have the right, but have they the *moral* right, to allow their children – be they mentally defective or not – to be used a human guinea-pigs?'

As in the book, Pappworth cited in his article those who shared his views on research ethics, lending weight to his argument and trying to prove to his antagonists that he was not alone. He quoted the eloquent and daring words of Sir Heneage Ogilvie, a leading surgeon at Guy's Hospital in London: 'What is new in medicine is research by fraud.' He even quoted the late Pope – Pius XII – whose pronouncements at a September 1958 conference were reproduced in *The Guardian*: 'Certain states show a tolerance difficult to understand concerning certain laboratory and clinical experiments... It is the observance of the moral order which gives a value and dignity to human action and which preserves a person's rectitude.'

Reference to a religious leader is not surprising, coming from a man of deep (albeit different) faith. Pappworth even uses religious language in the article, referring to the 'near-sanctity of the doctor-patient relationship', and, in his penultimate paragraph, placing himself in the ranks of those 'who believe in the sanctity of human life'. For him it was something of a holy war, as he called on those who shared his beliefs to 'fight a battle to defend the rights of all patients against the whims and ambitions of some doctors'.

Something that seems to have particularly distressed Pappworth was the diversion of excellent young doctors from the physician-friend role to the backrooms of research. 'The alarming position has been reached that when applying for a post as consultant physician a grain of research is considered the equal of a ton of clinical experience.'

Unlike the later book, 'Human Guinea Pigs: a Warning' named no names. Not only did Pappworth refrain from pointing the finger at individuals; he also decided not to reveal in which medical journals their reports had been published. His principal intention was to give information to a public that had little or no idea about what was happening in British medical research, and to get people talking. In this he undoubtedly succeeded – and he was prepared for the many fellow-doctors who mounted a counter-offensive.

The *BMJ* reviewed Pappworth's article on 27 October 1962, pointing out that for four or five years the Ethical Committee of the World Medical Association had already been studying the concerns he articulated. 'The subject is highly complex,' observed the anonymous reviewer. He cites the example of

William Withering, who investigated the effects of foxglove infusion on his dropsical patients. Without this trial, 'countless thousands of sufferers from heart disease would not have had the benefit of digitalis. These were experiments on human beings.' But he also recommends that Claude Bernard's *Introduction à l'Etude de la Médecine Experimentale* (of which Pappworth himself was a great admirer) 'should be read at least by those whose enthusiasm for investigation seems at times to run into conflict with their obligations as physicians in charge of patients... Hundreds and hundreds of experiments have [since] been conducted... which conflict with the principle of medical morality.' This balanced review by a medical professional suggests that Pappworth's article in a lay journal achieved its primary aim – to make people think.

Many doctors shared Pappworth's views on the danger of unregulated experimentation, and after the appearance of his article he was contacted by some. Most notably, Pappworth received a letter from Henry Beecher, Professor at the Harvard School of Medicine. In a 2012 article in *Annals of Internal Medicine,* Allan Gaw described Beecher and Pappworth as 'the two most prominent medical whistle-blowers in research ethics of the twentieth century', claiming that the letters they exchanged mark 'an important juncture in the genesis of modern clinical research ethics. Although they shared much in common, they differed radically in the strategies they adopted. Beecher chose to conceal the identities of individuals, whereas Pappworth believed that only by naming and shaming could any exposé act as a deterrent.'

Gaw argues that the letters gave each man that vital sense that he was not alone in his decision to publish the facts about dubious research practices. Beecher first wrote to Pappworth in response to 'Human Guinea Pigs: A Warning', describing 'an explosion... in research in man'. Three years later, in January 1965, he wrote to him again: 'I appreciate your detailed and thoughtful letter concerning our mutual interest... Certain elements in medicine in this country have long held the view that these problems must be swept under the rug. I do not at all agree with this point of view and I think that with the "explosion" just referred to, that these matters must be faced... It seems to me that a man must stand behind the work he publishes.'

In 1966, Beecher's article 'Ethics and Clinical Research' appeared in the *New England Journal of Medicine*. Twenty-two examples of what he considered to be unethical treatment of human research subjects were described. When, the following year, Pappworth published *Human Guinea Pigs* (an American edition appeared shortly afterwards), the author covered two hundred cases. 'Through these publications,' comments Gaw, 'Beecher and Pappworth blew the whistle on unethical clinical research and started a debate on research ethics that would continue for the next three decades.' As a professor at one of America's most prestigious medical schools, Beecher was a whistle-blower making a noise from within the establishment. Pappworth, meanwhile, was an outsider, a thorn in the flesh of the British medical hierarchy.

However, co-operation between the two whistle-blowers was not to last. In Pappworth's January 1965 letter, he first mooted the idea which was to bring to an end his correspondence with his transatlantic supporter. It was the issue of naming and shaming: 'What would your reaction be to a suggestion that summaries of some of the most offensive experiments be published together with the Journal references and names?' Beecher didn't respond for ten months, writing in November: 'While the individual who does it... must be severely criticized... I think someone has got to call attention to the problems as they exist'. Two months after this letter, in March 1965, Beecher presented a paper at a conference in Michigan which, as Gaw explains, 'cited specific examples of unethical research practice, but stopped short of giving names'. Meanwhile, in February Pappworth had announced in a letter to him: 'After much thought and great hesitation I have decided that I shall publish a book on Human Guinea Pigs with quotations, names and references to about 150 of the 500 odd questionable experiments of which I have details.'

Pappworth had agonised over his decision. But it remained one with which Beecher disagreed. His 1966 article in the *New England Journal of Medicine*, based on his Michigan paper, listed a host of articles proving that patients had been experimented on, sometimes at considerable risk to themselves and without their knowledge. Neither had consent been given against a background of clear explanations and hence informed decisions. But Beecher named no names.

Pappworth wanted to know why. Replying to his letter in July, Beecher explained: 'I discussed the matter with a senior Professor of Law at Harvard who assured me, as I had expected, that the investigators in these studies would, in many cases, be liable to criminal prosecution... My intention was to point to a widespread practice, not to individuals.' 'This,' states Gaw, 'was not good enough for Pappworth, and he responded immediately, questioning why Beecher had protected the guilty.'

Once again, Pappworth's priorities are illuminated: the patient comes first. If that means that the perpetrators of unethical research practices are brought before the law, so be it: it is not a doctor's job to collude in the whitewashing of his colleagues. But when, in the same letter, he asked Beecher to give him specific details of the references he had used, he found the drawbridge raised. On 29 July 1966, Beecher sent Pappworth what was to be the final letter in their correspondence: 'Everybody and his brother has been after me to divulge these names and at the time this paper went to press I decided that the only sensible way was to decline in all cases to give information not contained in the paper itself.'

And so Beecher retained his position as a respected figure at the heart of the American medical establishment while Pappworth, remaining on the edges, was in a better position to choose a more confrontational path. It was in his nature, after all. On 30 April 1967, just before the publication of *Human Guinea Pigs*, Pappworth wrote to Professor Desmond Laurence thanking him for sending him an as-yet unpublished Royal College of Physicians report on the ethical aspects of medical research. Ten days later Laurence responded: 'I have no doubt your 1962 article prepared people's minds for it, including mine.'

The *Twentieth Century* article certainly shook the medical world. Commenting on it in October 1962, the *BMJ*'s leading article remarked: 'The subject is highly complex and wide open to misinterpretation. If Jenner had not given the boy James Phipps cowpox and then subsequently attempted to give him smallpox the science of immunology would not have reached its position today'. The writer goes on to concede that there are many more examples, including those listed by Pappworth, 'to indicate that the physician's human obligations to his patients are sometimes abused'. The leader also touches on an argument close to Pappworth's heart: that 'editors should act as a check by refusing to publish some of the results of experiments on human beings'. And it does admit that, despite heated correspondence in the press and questions in Parliament, there has been little 'restraining' of 'those who cannot always understand the difference between guinea-pigs and human beings, especially when they are collected together in penitentiaries, reformatories, and institutions for the mentally defective'. Pappworth had certainly stirred debate. This pleased him; it also alarmed him, when he considered his position within British medicine. He remained a passionate but angry man.

Towards a public scandal

Whatever the opinions of the medical press, the national press seized on the topic with the gusto commonly employed whenever a good medical story breaks. In an article headed 'Doctors' Diagnosis', *The Times* of 18 October 1962 declared that Pappworth's article contained a 'serious charge that deserves a serious answer.' It pointed to the highlighting of 'the unpleasant and often dangerous experiments... frequently carried out on unsuspecting patients in hospitals'. Articles in the *Daily Express* and *The Guardian* also drew attention to the severity of Pappworth's claims.

So public interest continued, and Pappworth was able to reach his biggest audience yet by appearing on a television panel on 1 August 1963. The programme, part of a current-affairs series entitled *This Week*, was aired by ITV, Britain's only independent broadcasting channel at the time. To witness doctors debating a controversial topic was not something to which its audience was accustomed. Chaired by the well-known broadcaster Desmond Wilcox, the panel consisted of Helen Hodgson, founder of the Patients' Association, Dr Maurice Pappworth, and Dr Charles Fletcher of the Hammersmith Hospital and Postgraduate School of Medicine, who presented a popular medical programme called 'Your Life in Their Hands' Despite his television experience, Fletcher was clearly rattled by Pappworth's onslaught, and was even drawn into admitting that some young researchers 'do become indiscreet' – fodder for the following day's headlines. Pappworth was vigorously on the offensive, but as Helen Bamber observed, 'That was a very, very difficult situation for him. He had a family to protect. He had a lot to protect.'

Pappworth was introduced by Wilcox as a 'Harley Street consultant who exposed the practice of experiments on patients'. From the outset, Pappworth emphasised that there were those who shared his view: 'For many years a few doctors – including myself – have protested in medical journals strongly and at medical meetings against the ever increasingly common practice of doing experiments on patients without their valid consent.' Asked for an example, he tried to maximise his impact by the use of the second-person pronoun: 'You want to investigate shock. You do not wait for a patient who is in shock to be admitted to hospital – instead you produce shock in a patient.' He then went on to cite the case of twelve patients, including three teenagers, subjected to a particularly unpleasant heart procedure. It involved the insertion of a tube into the heart and then being deliberately tilted to induce shock – even though none of them suffered from heart disease, and so could not have gained any therapeutic benefit from the experiment. He also gave details of heart catheterization at the Hammersmith undertaken while a 'tightly fitting nose-clip' attached a mask to the patient's face. That mask and nose-clip were to play a recurrent villain's role in *Human Guinea Pigs*. Pappworth had evidently thought carefully beforehand about which examples in his armoury would strike the hardest.

Fletcher countered by adopting a sarcastic tone, insinuating wild exaggeration on Pappworth's part. He also resorted to below-the-belt tactics, such as referring to an appendectomy, 'which you I'm sure have never carried out.' He complained, as others were to do when Pappworth published his book four years later, of the 'emotional terms' in which his fellow panellist spoke. On a television programme on such a highly-charged subject, whoever had the stronger story to tell was bound to gain the upper hand. When Wilcox asked if it was possible that he might be admitted to hospital with a broken leg only to find that a piece of his liver had been removed during his stay, Pappworth's reply was immediate: 'Undoubtedly, and this is the trouble – and they would do so moreover under the guise of doing an investigation on you.'

This proved too much for Fletcher, who once more launched a cheap *ad hominem* attack. Turning to Pappworth, he enquired: 'Can I ask what hospital you're on the staff of?' Fletcher knew perfectly well that, as stated in Wilcox's introduction, Pappworth was a consultant operating out of his own independent practice. That senior London hospital post had never materialised. However he may have felt when Fletcher offered his taunt, Pappworth was later sufficiently recovered to hand-write a comment in the margin of the transcript: 'Lost his cool.'

Pappworth naturally steered the discussion to the question of informed consent. When pressed on his hospital's policy here, Fletcher tacked into a digression on diabetes, before eventually admitting that 'There are occasions when young research workers... do become so enthusiastic about the advance of knowledge that they do become indiscreet.' Pappworth's challenges about a research trial that had involved deliberately withholding insulin from diabetic patients, some of whom became comatose as a result, was countered by Fletcher: 'The person was young and enthusiastic at the time and should be forgiven.' So he handed to Pappworth – and to the press – a quotation that did nothing to help his cause.

From the Severall's Hospital in Chichester, Russell Barton wrote to Pappworth the day after the programme: 'Many congratulations on your brilliant performance last night. I liked the crack about which hospital do you work at. I think it is a dreadful reflection on the teaching system in this country that the number one teacher of clinical medicine has not a teaching hospital appointment.' A letter the following month from Anthony Wilkinson of Associated Rediffusion, producers of This Week, informed Pappworth that the programme had generated a large amount of correspondence. It was Pappworth's first television appearance, and he seemed to have made a success of it. The small Jewish Liverpudlian knew instinctively, it seemed, how to blossom on screen.

But whatever the response from like-minded doctors and journalists, that from the medical journals came through gritted teeth. After publication of the *Twentieth Century* article and his appearance on *This Week*, Pappworth's difficulties in having correspondence published in the medical press intensified. At the end of August 1963, the assistant editor of the *BMJ*, J.R. Wilson, wrote to him maintaining that 'a time does come when further correspondence does not very much help'. At the beginning of September, Wilson informed Pappworth that the subject of experimentation on man had enjoyed 'a very thorough airing... Every correspondence has to come to an end some time.'

From polemic to publication

The article paved the way for publication of Pappworth's book. On 18 October 1962, the left-wing publisher Victor Gollancz, whom Pappworth had recently met at a party, wrote to him: 'I have just read the "piece" in The *Guardian* about your article in *Twentieth Century*. I found your material quite horrifying, and am writing to ask whether you would contemplate writing a short book, either exclusively on this subject, or combining it with other cognate material.' Pappworth responded positively, and just over a week later discussed the book proposal with Gollancz's daughter Livia. Writing back to Pappworth that day, Gollancz was already setting out details of an advance, royalty payments, and the publisher/author split in the case of a paperback edition and serialisation (about both of which Gollancz was optimistic). In a postscript he added that 'your earnings might be considerable'. Stipulating that the book should be between 60,000 and 70,000 words, he makes it clear that he would like the manuscript to be delivered as soon as possible.

For a man prolix both in his written and spoken words, that 70,000 ceiling was always going to be difficult, as was the request for early delivery: Dr Pappworth was a busy man. But the opportunity to have this cause so close to his heart published by a highly-respected publisher who shared his views was one he wasn't going to turn down.

In March 1963 – less than six months after Gollancz's initial letter to Pappworth – his daughter Livia reminded their author that his manuscript was due round about the end of the month. Mid-April was agreed as a delivery date, but a letter dated 9 May shows that Miss Gollancz was still waiting. It is scarcely surprising that Pappworth was struggling to complete the work on time. The pressure he was under, despite subsequent editing, does still show in the sometimes sloppy structure of the book. It was certainly a factor in the turn of events at Victor Gollancz Ltd. Having finally received the manuscript and sent it to a reader for comment, Gollancz wrote to Pappworth on 26 July 1963 that 'I am awfully sorry to have to tell you that we cannot publish Human Guinea Pigs in anything like its present form. The real point is, to put it bluntly, it just isn't, in its present form, a book.'

Gollancz suggested two possibilities. First, that Pappworth should 'enlist the aid of a literary or journalistic friend to assist in rewriting and reshaping the whole thing. For this purpose, we should of course be happy to send you the three reports we have had.' However, 'If you feel that this would involve too much time and to be too speculative, then, without publishing the manuscript, we should of course pay you the £350 provided for in the contract. I am terribly sorry about this.'

Gollancz was embarrassed. Pappworth was furious – and deeply upset. As he explained to Livia Gollancz, 'I was pressed for time when I wrote my book and was very conscious of the fact that it would require some rewriting and condensation, especially of the second part. But I thought that a firm of your repute would help with this, and am very surprised by your completely negative attitude.'

Pappworth had by this stage read the main reader's report which Gollancz had forwarded to him. The report is indeed fairly damning: 'For obvious reasons Dr. Pappworth uses quotations as much as possible in his argument and this makes for an extremely disjointed account. The writing is often very muddled but, in my opinion, Part I could be made into a consecutively readable section if it were drastically edited.' On the 'case-histories' described in Part II, the verdict is that they 'become terribly monotonous in their sameness' and so 'readability vanishes…. Occasionally, the author draws a conclusion (or makes a snyde [sic] remark) at the end of a case-history', although they 'are all quite horrifying enough to make their own points unaided.'

While conceding that the 'theme of Dr Pappworth's book is extremely important,' the reader insists that 'in its present form the book itself seems to me so inadequate as to be likely to do harm rather than good'. It does not take much effort to imagine how Pappworth must have felt on reading this indictment. However, he retained sufficient spirit to pencil in the margin alongside this last point, 'Harm to whom?' He was to grow used to another of the criticisms in the report – that of the 'over-emotional' tone he chose at times to use. Against the reader's comment that the author 'makes a mistake in not presenting the case of his opponents – his failure to do so reinforces the impression that his attack in not sufficiently supported by facts and logic,' Pappworth scribbles 'So stupid.'

The report continues: 'The second part, with its hundreds of baldly reported, technically worded case histories, I found virtually unreadable, and feel that it would be so to the great majority of laymen.' Given that the version of *Human Guinea Pigs* eventually published went out of its way to explain technical terms to the lay reader, Pappworth was evidently absorbing some of the criticism. Approaching the end of his report, the reader declares: 'What is wanted is not editing as much as a complete rewriting, and whether Dr Pappworth has sufficient literary experience for the purpose seems to me doubtful.' The report concludes by describing Pappworth's approach as 'obsessional', and suspects that 'he is grossly exaggerating the menace... It is not at all a *persuasive* book, and it becomes very dull as a result of repetition.'

Once Gollancz had decided to reject the book, his tone in correspondence becomes harsh and inflexible. The businessman has taken over from the publishing visionary. Should Pappworth find another publisher, Gollancz insists that he should reimburse his company the £350 which he had offered to pay the author when he turned the book down in March. It was at this point that Pappworth withdrew from his association with Victor Gollancz Ltd, telling Livia in September that 'I am willing to release you from your obligation'. The letter is short, the tone dignified.

Pappworth wasn't going to throw in the towel. Having worked so hard to produce his manuscript, he was determined to find a publisher. In all, three publishers hung onto the manuscript for several months, before finally rejecting it on the advice of libel lawyers. A letter to him by Graham C Greene of Jonathan Cape on 23 November 1964, more than a year and a half after *Human Guinea Pigs* was turned down by Gollancz, indicates that Cape now had the manuscript 'under very active consideration'. While Cape was still reading it, the libel report on *Human Guinea Pigs* was completed. Dated 8 January 1965, it was drawn up by libel expert Michael Rubinstein (who was, incidentally, a close neighbour of Pappworth's). Writing to his neighbour on 17 December 1964, Rubinstein assured him that he was happy to read the book for libel, 'all the more so because knowing you I am quite sure it will be fascinating.' A letter to Pappworth three weeks later shows that Rubinstein had finished *Human Guinea Pigs*, which he read 'with horrified fascination throughout'.

Rubinstein found little in the manuscript that could give rise to a libel action, given that (a point emphasised in *Human Guinea Pigs*) all accounts of experiments had already been written up in medical journals. He did warn Pappworth that he 'could be shown to have inaccurately referred to, quoted or condensed the published reports'. Rubinstein continues: 'More seriously, the cases where patients experimented on are stated to have died (or other especially harmful or unpleasant consequences followed any experiment) might involve imputations (under the law of this country) of manslaughter at least, against those responsible for the deaths'. Rubinstein notes two instances when 'the experiment you criticise may involve criminal offences of fraud and common assault', which entails 'an unquestioned libel upon all those listed as having carried out experiments in the manner you criticise throughout the book'.

Two pages of the report consist of Rubinstein's advice on 'the expressions you use which might be taken to indicate an emotional rather than wholly rational and logical or, better, objective attitude'. Here we find the *leitmotif* of many views on Pappworth's rhetoric. In his marginal annotations, we can see that Pappworth followed most of Rubinstein's advice, cutting or changing many of the inflammatory phrases, or those which might be challenged.

At the end of his copy of the libel report, Pappworth scribbles a summarising sentence. His note flags up an important development since the rejection by Gollancz. Recognising that *Human Guinea Pigs* was less well written than *A Primer of Medicine*, Helen Bamber enlisted the help of her friend, the writer Stuart Smith, to help Pappworth in editing his manuscript. Having got his material down on paper – a process which Bamber describes as 'terribly painful for him' – Pappworth was loath to revisit it. Stuart Smith's editorial assistance was just what he needed. How to make a manuscript on a specialist subject more accessible to the general reader, and therefore more marketable? His struggle to get it right is a telling case study.

The book did remain under serious consideration by Jonathan Cape. By mid-June 1965, Graham C Greene – Cape's managing director, and nephew of the novelist Graham Greene – was able to offer Pappworth a contract and was 'actively pursuing the question of libel insurance'. Discussions and amendments continued for a further four months until, on 20 October, Greene wrote to Pappworth advising him that his typescript would be returned to him by the publisher's van driver. In a postscript, Greene asked him to return the draft contract. Once again, it had all come to nothing.

Human Guinea Pigs was at this stage also being assessed by Cassell Publishers. Pappworth had been assured by Cassell's senior editor Kenneth Parker of their 'very great interest in the subject, and our willingness to do all we can to achieve publication'. Cassell did not exactly haggle, but they certainly proved unwilling to publish on Pappworth's conditions. A cocktail of legal advice and – so Pappworth suspected – interference by the medical branch of Cassell's publishing empire led to their decision in March 1966 to decline *Human Guinea Pigs*.

Pappworth, bitterly disappointed, and lapsing into his vocabulary's danger zone, accused the company of trying to exert censorship. Parker's response was curt and bruising. Describing Pappworth's letter as 'incorrect in every respect,' he asserted that 'The only censorship we acknowledge outside that of our own choice is that imposed by the Official Secrets Act.' There is something patronising about that final sentence.

On 25 March 1966 Pappworth admitted to Helen Bamber, 'I am back to square one now but definitely determined to publish.' Interest in the topic continued. At the beginning of that year, Adam Raphael had written an article for the *Guardian* headlined 'Unconscious Pioneers'. Drawing attention to the dangers outlined in Pappworth's *Twentieth Century* article. Raphael's piece was carefully filed away by the publishers Routledge & Kegan Paul. The subject remained in the public eye: a letter from Charles Roger of the *Sunday Mirror*, in mid-April, asked if he could read the manuscript with a view to serialising *Human Guinea Pigs*.

Pappworth continued to receive advice from his lawyer and friend, Harry Sacker. In a letter dated 10 June, Sacker admitted that his 'first concern' was 'the possibility that there might be accidental libel, e.g., an incorrect reference whereby the performance of an experiment by A was attributed to B... if there were such a libel you and the publishers would be jointly liable for damages.' Sacker was also worried by 'proof of malice': might one of the researchers condemned in *Human Guinea Pigs* come forward as a plaintiff? This was disconcerting territory for Pappworth. The expert diagnostician must have realised that his condition as a whistle-blower threatened not life but livelihood. Sacker warns his client that 'Insurance by authors is unusual and underwriters would naturally be suspicious,' and the premium high. 'As I see it your reputation would be as much at stake in any libel proceedings as would that of the plaintiff'. Nearly a year earlier, Rubinstein had advised Pappworth that 'the market for libel insurance is so restricted and exclusive' that probably 'no Underwriters will be prepared to take the risk.'

But in summer 1966, Pappworth did succeed in finding a publisher. The contract came from Routledge and Kegan Paul, whose editorial director Norman Franklin was willing to take the risk, and eager to publish a book which he anticipated generating much publicity and plenty of sales. At the end of March, Pappworth had submitted the typescript to Norman's brother and colleague, Colin. Tellingly, he adds: 'I do not want you to submit it to *any medical* for opinion', concluding, 'Let's hope the third time will be lucky.' In a letter dated 27 April 1966 and enclosing a draft contract (with the author paid £100 on signature), Franklin tells Pappworth that 'We feel that it is our duty to publish this book, and would like to put it across as effectively as we can; we are not quite clear whether it will have a general market but certainly it should achieve maximum publicity.' Publication was planned for 'the very beginning of 1967', although in the event it did not appear until May. Franklin continues: 'I look forward to a real stink when it comes, and rely on you not being camera shy, but eager to meet the press.'

Recognising that the typescript would need close editing, Routledge advertised in the *New Statesman* for someone who could work on the book at home, and received a response from a Miss Kathleen Orr. Orr's handwritten notes, sent to the publisher in early August 1966, reveal that she did a very competent editing job. 'It seems to me,' she remarked, 'that even the most sympathetic and interested reader might be overwhelmed by the constant repetition of similar activities, e.g. cardiac catheterisation... I have therefore made a short list of suggested experiments to cut out but would like it explained to Dr Pappworth that these have been selected because of their low interest value rather than their medical import.' In a later letter to Colin Franklin, Miss Orr admits that 'I shall certainly be very wary if any of my family ever visit a teaching hospital!'

Human Guinea Pigs, with the subtitle *Experimentation on Man*, was published in May 1967. Routledge billed it in the BBC magazine *The Listener* as 'Dr M.H. Pappworth's startling report'. It was priced at 32 shillings – in contemporary money, £1.60, but around £27 adjusted for inflation. An American edition was published early the following year by the Beacon Press, Boston. At the beginning of August 1967, Routledge exchanged contracts with Penguin for a paperback edition.

Like almost every author, Pappworth felt that his book could be selling better; like almost every author, he wrote to his publisher with complaints and suggestions. In a letter to Norman Franklin on 16 June 1967, he wrote that 'The sales are extremely disappointing, especially when the amount of publicity in press, radio and television is considered. May not the lack of sales be due to lack of advertising?' He had been doing the detective work familiar to all writers trying to track their new baby's progress: 'The Times Bookshop has a display window of recent books and inside the shop has a similar table display. I have been in the shop three times in the past three weeks but have never seen a copy of my book on show.'

In an article on medical ethical committees for *World Medicine* in 1978, Pappworth explained that some of the contents of *Human Guinea Pigs* had been leaked ('not by me') prior to publication – chiefly because of the delays in finding a publisher. This leakage made Pappworth vulnerable to those implicated in his accusations. In a much later article, for the *BMJ* in 1990, he revealed that he had at this time received three anonymous calls from men claiming to be senior physicians and urging him 'for the good of the profession' not to publish the book. Such back-handed pressure, delivered in this sinister way, was of course unsettling, but made him all the more determined to fight the establishment. I have no recollection of his ever discussing these anonymous telephone calls with his family.

But Pappworth was never a lone voice in the wilderness. There were plenty who supported him – even if they were not often willing to voice this support in public. In a private letter to Pappworth in March 1966, Henry Beecher of Harvard declared that 'I am not at all surprised that some doctors opposed your publication. I do not think that is adequate reason for silence on your part. I wish you luck.' Luck, courage, and a very dense hide: he was going to need all these in the year ahead.

Chapter Six

The whistle blows: the book and the storm

'From inability to let well alone, from too much zeal for the new, and contempt for what is old; from putting knowledge before wisdom, science before art, cleverness before common sense; from treating patients as cases; and from making "the cure" of the disease more grievous than the endurance of the same, Good Lord deliver us.'

(Sir Robert Hutchison, Scottish physician and paediatrician, quoted in Maurice Pappworth's 'Human Guinea Pigs')

Respect and consent: the red lines of research

To hold in his hand the solid 228-page hardback of this, the most hard-fought achievement of his life so far, was a moment of personal triumph for Maurice Pappworth. He was fifty-seven, an age when many people are looking forward to running on fewer cylinders in their work. But this was a new kind of beginning. Delight, surging up from some deep place inside their father that they rarely saw, was not how his three daughters remember that all-important moment. We were probably more interested in the release of The Beatles' album Sgt. Pepper's Lonely Hearts Club Band a couple of weeks later, on 1 June. There was plenty of anxiety: the big question now was how public, press and professionals were going to respond to this most controversial of books.

Routledge's cover designer had chosen a mustard yellow for the dustjacket, with plain lettering and no artwork – not the sort of look which would encourage you to pick it up from a bookshop display. By contrast, the Italian edition, *Cavie Humane,* was striking and colourful; the US edition featured a dramatic large white syringe slanting down the front, with a royal blue dustjacket and green lettering. Readers of the German edition, *Menschen als Versuchskaninchen*, published in 1968, were treated to a photograph of four doctors in white gowns, headgear and masks, the patient invisible. The Pelican edition, published two years after the hardback, was to feature a ward full of beds, with the covers of just one bed turned back – a sinister indication that its former occupant is now in the research laboratory.

As Charlie Gibbs has pointed out in his 2010 dissertation for the University of Kent on 'The Genesis and Impact of *Human Guinea Pigs* on Medical Ethics during the 1960s and 1970s', Maurice Pappworth was the right person to publish this book, as 'an outsider to the established medical scene in Britain'. Thus he felt able to conduct 'sustained attacks on some fellow physicians and their approaches to medical research'. 'At the heart of his assertions,' Gibbs maintains, 'is the idea that... there should be greater checks and balances... [and that] individual doctors should take ultimate responsibility for their clinical research.' One soon realises, Gibbs concludes, that 'objectivity is not one of Pappworth's major concerns'.

If objectivity were not one of Pappworth's chief concerns in *Human Guinea Pigs*, what did he aim to achieve in writing the book? On one of its first pages, Pappworth claims that 'The main purpose of this book is to show that the ethical problems arising from human experimentation have become one of the cardinal issues of our time'. Pappworth continues: 'I believe that only by frank discussion among informed people, lay as well as medical, can a solution be reached.'

His determination to reach out to the lay reader meant that Pappworth explained some of the many technical terms necessary in such a work, and tried to make the material as accessible as he could to the non-professional: 'I am fully aware of the fact that lay people may find the accounts of some of the experiments difficult to follow... but hope that the general gist of what the experiments involve will be obtained from the necessarily brief summaries.' Pappworth advises the reader to consult the diagrams of the human body's circulation drawn by his wife Jean, a talented artist, and reproduced at the front of the book.

Pappworth hopes 'that the ends of research may be effectively served without any of the harm done at present'. That advances such as the treatment of diabetes with insulin and the introduction of penicillin have been the result of research means it is especially important that these great success stories are not used as an excuse for lax ethical standards. Ever mindful of how medicine and cruelty may suddenly collide, he aims to champion the vulnerable, especially babies and children, who 'call for more consideration than other groups'. A child cannot, of course, give consent to take part in an experimental procedure, but it was believed by many at this time that as long as both parents consented, that was sufficient.

However, as Pappworth points out, 'the law both here and in America appears to be very definite, namely, that parents... cannot give valid legal consent to any action that is not for the immediate benefit of the child concerned'. Pappworth also sought to protect those to whom (as was normal at the time) he referred as 'mental defectives and the mentally sick'. Was such a person *capable* of giving consent? he wonders. A further difficulty is the pressure to volunteer to undergo an experiment, which he describes as 'enormous'. It could be argued that every hospital inpatient was, potentially, at risk. At the time he was gathering evidence, many people stayed in hospital for up to six weeks, thus presenting perfect fodder for experimentation.

And there are the prisoners: in the United States, it was common practice after the war to use those in penitentiaries as experimental fodder. In return, the prisoner might receive payment, a box of cigarettes or early parole. Pappworth believed that the British could not afford to be complacent about the absence of prisoner experimentation: 'we have evidence of a clear desire on the part of some experimenters to use criminals in this way'. He quotes the principal medical officer of the Distillers' Company (the UK manufacturer, it will be remembered, of the infamous drug Thalidomide) recommending the use of criminals to test drug toxicity. Pappworth also cites a 1944 experiment in a Chicago prison and a New Jersey reformatory – an attempt to 'try out new cures' for malaria by deliberately infecting the subjects. All volunteers were required to sign a document whose final paragraph ran: 'I hereby certify that this offer is made voluntarily and without compulsion. I have been instructed that if my offer is accepted I shall be entitled to remuneration amounting to… dollars.' There is, surely, a lingering scent of corruption here.

Pappworth's objectives also include a reminder that 'Non-Patient Volunteers' face difficulties and dangers. In this group he includes medical and nursing students, junior doctors and other hospital staff, all of whom may be subject to 'a degree of coercion being exerted by the experimenter'. For the prospective volunteer is 'often in some way dependent on him'. He might, for example, be a student, anxious that 'he will reduce himself in his professor's eyes if he refuses… Or he may feel that he can gain favour by coming forward promptly.'

Pappworth suggests that all hospital staff, both clinical and support, should always be approached in a group when volunteers were being sought, and never individually. 'If a student is approached individually by his professor he may find it very embarrassing to refuse.' He also recommends that students or nurses under twenty-one should participate only if written consent from their parents is obtained, pointing out that that the age at which consent to treatment may be accepted as valid 'has never been settled in the English courts'. Doctors and nurses, whether fully qualified or still in training, are naturally all too well aware of the risks they might be undertaking should they participate in an experiment, however well directed.

What particularly worried Pappworth was that patients might easily confuse therapeutic experimentation with research for research's sake. A patient 'could simply be allowed to think that what he is undergoing is part of the investigations for which he entered hospital... The fact that what is being done is an experiment quite unrelated to the patient's own disease or condition is frequently not revealed to him at all.'

From Part Two of *Human Guinea Pigs*, entitled *Principles*, one may gain a very clear sense of Pappworth's objectives. He wasn't simply out to shock, expose and scare; he wanted things to be done – not just an open admission of what had been going on in hospitals, but also practical solutions in the form of safeguards, ethical codes and legislation. He describes the primary function of these as 'to adjust the balance of power so as to protect the patient or client against the practitioner who has the immense advantages which are derived from knowledge and experience'. As always, Pappworth sets himself up as the advocate of the weak and vulnerable against the powerful and strong. He was a champion of the underdog, indeed – but fully aware that also in need of protection are conscientious doctors themselves, who might otherwise suffer 'exploitation by the black sheep' prepared to defy ethical codes.

Pappworth was fearless because he felt so secure in his ethics: these determined and guided his professional life. In a sub-section, 'Proposed Codes Concerning Human Experimentation', he reminds the reader that 'The best-known ethical code governing doctor-patient relationships is that of Hippocrates... who expressed the view that the profession of medicine could not survive without a sound moral philosophy, and formulated his famous oath.' Pappworth had his own suggestions for a code governing human experimentation, which 'would be concerned with the following principles: equality; valid consent; prohibited subjects; previous animal experiments; experimenters' competence; proper records'.

On 'the principle of equality' he is especially eloquent, for it chimed with central tenets of his Jewish faith: 'No experiments should be contemplated, proposed or undertaken to which, if he were in circumstances identical to those of the intended subjects, the experimenter would even hesitate to submit himself or members of his own family, or anybody for whom he had any respect or affection. This principle of equality should be the cornerstone of the whole edifice of any code. It is essentially a restatement of the Golden Rule... preached by Jesus and the advice given by Rabbi Hillel a hundred years earlier, "Do not unto any man that which you would not have done to yourself."'

The 'prohibited subjects' on which experimentation should under no circumstances be undertaken include, according to Pappworth, the mentally sick, and the elderly or dying. Experiments on these categories 'must be indefensible if we take the principle of equality and valid consent seriously'. Pappworth concedes that 'Perhaps a case could be made out for the use of prison inmates [in Britain], provided there was valid consent and proper terms of compensation were included in a contract. But,' he continues, 'to subject prison inmates to procedures which may injure them is a cheap trick played on men who are taking their punishment.' And so he concludes: 'Prison inmates, then, are a group on whom no experiments should be performed.'

Pappworth is on less controversial grounds when he writes about having witnessed the trial use of new cancer treatments 'where the suffering produced by the agent in question has been very much worse than the suffering caused by the disease itself... The use of patients who are dying as subjects for experiments is shocking and wrong. This should hardly need saying... Where a patient cannot be saved, it is common humanity that he should be allowed to die in peace.'

Here was a doctor very interested in legal as well as moral matters. He corresponded on ethical issues with Immanuel (later Lord) Jakobovits, who became Chief Rabbi of Great Britain and the Commonwealth, and whose books included *Jewish Medical Ethics* (1959) and *Jewish Law Faces Modern Problems* (1965). Among his close friends there were probably more lawyers than doctors, and a section in Part Two of *Human Guinea Pigs* is devoted to 'Legal Considerations'. Here, he argued that medical research, 'like all activities in our society, is subject to common-law principles of general applicability'. Analysing the legal position in 1967, Pappworth considered 'that some legislation is needed for the responsible and conscientious experimenter'.

Can a form signed by a sick patient necessarily be classed as genuinely valid consent? The ambiguity here meant that, in the case of an accident, the researcher might be liable to 'prosecution for assault or trespass'. This, for Pappworth, was one of many reasons why stronger rules should be put in place. They could offer protection all round – as they already did for experimentation on animals. Every year, he informs us, Her Majesty's Stationery Office publishes a very detailed account of vivisection experiments. 'I seriously advocate that a similar list be published of all experiments done on hospital patients, giving full details of the nature and purpose of each experiment.'

Accountability depends on documentation; so Pappworth also insists that proper records should be kept by experimenters and *'included in the patient's records'*. He not unreasonably points out that 'what has been done to him is virtually part of his medical history… Quite often, when a complication does occur, repeated or different side-effects can appear much later.' With this in mind, he goes on to 'advocate legislation to make it compulsory for all doctors to report all deaths and major complications directly and indirectly due to any experimental investigation to a central bureau at the Ministry of Health, and that severe penalties be instituted for ignoring this order.' Although Pappworth lists six possible objections that might be raised to ethical codes, they are mentioned only to be dismissed. As we shall see, the official line was that these things couldn't be legislated, and should be left to the doctor's clinical judgment.

But according to Pappworth, 'whether or not any proposed experiment is legally and ethically justifiable must never be the sole opinion and decision of the experimenter himself or his team, but must always be the decision of properly constituted consultation committees'. Here we see the emergence of a key outcome of *Human Guinea Pigs*: the ethical committee. 'Each large hospital or, preferably, hospital group must have a committee of doctors, but one member must be a clinician who himself is not engaged in any research and there should be at least one lay member, preferably but not necessarily a lawyer. In Britain each Regional Hospital Board [an earlier version of current Hospital Trusts] would have such a committee' – though he concedes that the teaching hospitals would wish to maintain their independence.

Pappworth had evidently thought through in minute detail the procedures for initiating and running these committees. All this from a man who made no secret of being bored by committees and who avoided, wherever possible, finding himself on one. 'In Britain each research committee should be responsible to the General Medical Council… [which] in its turn would be answerable to Parliament.' The committees would be responsible for deciding whether or not proposed experiments should be undertaken. Where an experiment was allowed to go ahead, the committee would be given a full report from the doctors who conducted it. Pappworth, always with an eye on the detail, then proceeded to list all the information which should be included in the report. The Medical Research Committees' reports should be sent to 'a central registry office, which should annually publish a brief summary of all human experiments undertaken as is now done in Britain for animal experiments'.

These are all sensible, practical suggestions, and it can be fairly argued that Pappworth's proposals regarding legislation, accountability, transparency and a system of checks and balances were a chief motivation behind his writing the book. However, another possible reason for *Human Guinea Pigs* was that Pappworth quite simply had an axe to grind about the regrettable direction in which, in his view, post-war British medicine seemed to be moving. He believed that 'a certain amount' of medical research and its subsequent reporting in the professional journals was driven by 'the personal ambition of the doctor' more than by any 'real desire to help medicine itself'. The published reports of experiments were a particular bugbear: 'If medical editors themselves refused to publish papers which did not furnish evidence that the experiments they reported had been carried out in terms of the principles suggested, then the knowledge that the account of an unjustifiable experiment would not be published would, I believe, give considerable pause to those about to embark on such an experiment.'

In his conclusion, Pappworth includes a section called 'Real Volunteers'. He proposes that research workers might appeal, 'publicly and openly', for real volunteers, with clear explanations of the purpose of the experiment and the risks involved. He states that he has no objections, 'within certain limits', to paying the 'real volunteers' provided certain safeguards are met. This is what happens now. A poster campaign aimed at recruiting volunteers to participate in flu research was conspicuous on the London Underground during the winter of 2015-16: the payment offered was £2,500.

Case-notes: the chronicles of cruelty

The experiments cited in the book had generally taken place over the ten years prior to its publication and were conducted mostly in Britain, the United States and Canada. The British examples came almost exclusively from teaching hospitals.

To objections that he cited more American than British cases (125 out of 260 altogether), Pappworth in the paperback edition pointed out that he was able to include only a fraction of the reports he had read. As in the UK alone there were 162 medical journals and six thousand such journals published worldwide (over two million pages, he assures us), he obviously couldn't read them all. Most of the British experiments he cited took place at the Hammersmith Hospital – partly because it was at this time the Postgraduate Medical School of London. Pappworth clearly felt that the mantra of this institution then was that the end justifies the means, and the researcher is always in complete control of the situation – a view that he dismissed as 'arrogant'.

He certainly describes some horrific procedures which will make the reader wince with empathetic pain. The detail in which he writes about, for example, cardiac catheterization, is not for the faint-hearted. We have given some examples in the Introduction, and this chapter will not reel off an exhaustive list of ethically dubious research procedures. It aims instead to try to identify his reasons for selecting them.

Part One of *Human Guinea Pigs* is called 'What is Being Done'. Here Pappworth focuses on certain categories of 'human guinea pig', almost all of whom are particularly vulnerable: infants and children, pregnant women, 'mental defectives and the mentally sick', prison inmates, the dying and the old, the experimenters themselves, patients awaiting operations, and patients as controls. He uses some effective props: what seems particularly likely to distress and frighten, especially when inflicted on children, is the frequent fitting of tight face masks and nose clips to monitor breathing during experiments, or to instil potentially harmful gases.

As we have seen, Pappworth details experiments performed on newborn babies and young children, and on pregnant women – some of them teenagers. He highlights unpleasant and invasive procedures practised on cardiac and cancer patients. Pappworth's polemic is rich with warnings and leading questions. He informs the reader, for example, that an injection doesn't always end up in the right place: during a research procedure (as in therapeutic treatment) a contrast medium, a substance to enhance visibility, might be accidentally injected into a main liver artery or the left renal artery. He asks whether informed consent was obtained in every case: most of the reports do not specify. In the 1969 paperback edition, Pappworth reveals that, since first publication of the book, he has had many conversations with doctors on the subject of consent. From them he learnt that many experimental physicians merely told a patient that a tube or catheter was to be inserted into the blood vessel of his arm and/or leg. But what they failed to disclose was that the catheter would then be passed 'far beyond its point of insertion – for example along the femoral artery, through the abdominal aorta and thoracic aorta and finally into the heart'. Had he known such details in full, would the patient have given his consent?

Pappworth's descriptions of experiments carried out on patients with liver and blood diseases are based on 1960 reports by researchers, including Professor Sheila Sherlock, at the Hammersmith Hospital. In an experiment at the Hammersmith two years earlier, intended to measure heart output, subjects were given cardiac catheterization and intravenous infusion of a radioactive substance, with a wide-bore needle kept in the main artery and the application of the infamous face mask and nose clip. Pappworth tells us that the technique was first tried out on four anaesthetised dogs 'and then (the comparison of numbers is important) on eighty-six un-anaesthetised adults'. None of the subjects was already suffering from cardiac failure or leaking valves, so the experiment cannot have been of any therapeutic value to them.

One of Pappworth's postgraduate students told him how he had witnessed in the United States a very complex cardiac catheterization carried out on a cash-strapped student who was paid for volunteering. During the experiment he developed 'profound shock and collapse, followed by stoppage of the heart. He was successfully brought back to life, having for a few moments been virtually dead. The experimenter then *continued with the experiment as though nothing had happened*. The experimenter's true attitude to his subject seems to have been expressed in the remark he made to those present at this performance: "He must be a fool to repeatedly come back to us."' So the poor, who return to take part once more in hazardous experiments in order to make some money, may be added to the Pappworth catalogue of the vulnerable.

He is also graphic when describing how prisoners in the United States were infected with the plague and beri-beri. As they have almost identical diets, sleeping hours and daily routines, prisoners can prove very useful as subjects in controlled clinical trials. Pappworth identified these inmates as vulnerable, because their situation had turned them into victims of bribery. 'The reduction of sentence in prison under the parole system is viewed as a reward for good conduct. Service as a subject in a medical experiment is considered to be a form of good conduct': hence the lure of early parole or other bonuses offered to those willing to participate in research. In an article in July 1963, *Time* magazine claimed that the US government was sponsoring medical research in fifteen penal institutions. In return for submitting to experiments, the article stated, federal prisoners were given rewards ranging from a packet of cigarettes to twenty-five dollars in cash. In Oklahoma State Penitentiary, the medical director made deals with pharmaceutical companies to test out their new drugs on prisoners. 'For volunteering as subjects for these tests the prisoners received small fees. The doctors grossed an estimated three hundred thousand dollars a year.'

In the Pelican paperback edition, Pappworth goes on to discuss 'Definitions of Death', 'Consent of Donors and Donors' Relatives', 'Consent of Recipient', 'The Likely Success of Transplants', 'Donor and Recipient Selection', 'National Pride and Transplants', 'Financial and Economic Aspects of Transplants', and 'Some Further Points about Transplants'. He was right up to the wire here, presumably writing this section as the book was about to go to press. He worried that transplant surgeons were, in the midst of all the excitement at these new developments, failing to take the public into their confidence. (The first human heart transplants had taken place in December 1967.) With the advances in medical science, ethical and practical issues were more relevant than ever.

Challengingly tough though it was, Pappworth's litany of abuses in *Human Guinea Pigs* did not come unsupported by a carefully tailored strategy. Pappworth could appear perfectly reasonable (he was, after all, a scientist, trained to abjure the tall story). He was even prepared to admit, towards the end of the book, that since the First World War patients' status had improved – for example the requirement (dating from 1914) that written consent be obtained before an operation is performed.

So he seizes his chance: informed consent in the case of experimentation, he argues, should be the natural sequel. Given the £16 million of public money spent on medical research in the financial year 1962-63, should not the taxpayer, through laws enacted by Parliament, 'have a say in the way that this part of his money is spent?' We must remember that his book was aimed at the lay reader as much as the medical professional, and the 'taxpayers' money!' rallying cry has always proved effective. His call for 'Real Volunteers' may be seen partly as an attempt to avoid the anti-progress smear. Pappworth did not wish to be seen as someone who was prepared to throw the baby out with the bathwater, and continued to insist that he recognised the need for medical research.

Wherever possible, he introduced the opinions of those who agreed with him – the more authoritative the better. He quoted Pope Pius XII, who in September 1952 declared that the patient has an obligation *not* to run undue risks as an experimental subject. He naturally brought in Henry Beecher: 'Any clarification of human experimentation as "for the good of society" is to be viewed with distaste, even alarm... Such high-flown expressions... have been used within living memory as cover for outrageous ends.' Pappworth quoted an eminent surgeon from Guy's Hospital in London, Sir William Heneage Ogilvie, who, writing in *The Lancet* in 1952, warned, 'The science of experimental medicine is something new and sinister; for it is capable of destroying in our minds the old faith that we, the doctors, are the servants of the patients whom we have undertaken to care for, and, in the minds of the patients, the complete trust that they can place their lives or the lives of their loved ones in our care.' Pappworth was without doubt very good at identifying eloquent endorsers of his principles.

A favourite of his was Dr Otto Guttentag of the University of California Medical School, already mentioned as the inventor of the 'physician-friend' concept. He remarked – approvingly quoted by Pappworth – that 'Theirs is the relationship between two I's... "the mutual obligation of two equals."' He also cited Guttentag's 1953 article in *Science*, which included the warning, 'Experimentation on the hopelessly sick requires a terrific amount of self-criticism, self-discipline, and understanding of life's essential attributes, lest it be perverted to unconscious barbarity.'

Pappworth referred to S.E. Stumpf, of the Department of Philosophy at Nashville's Vanderbilt University. In *Annals of Internal Medicine* in 1966, Stumpf observed that 'Modern medicine has provoked some serious moral questions, not through malignant perversity, but because of the enormous momentum medical science has gained in the past few decades.' This point underlines so much of the significance of *Human Guinea Pigs*: with medicine developing at such a rate, it was more essential than ever to establish codes of conduct governing professional practice.

Another of Pappworth's strategies was simply to allow the experimenters, in their published accounts, to speak for themselves, as in the report of the 1961 experiment on 'mentally deficient' infants in Boston quoted in the Introduction. In *Annals of Surgery*, 1950, experimenters at Johns Hopkins Hospital in Baltimore gave details of a particularly invasive catheter penetration. 'There have been no serious complaints,' insist the authors of the report. 'However, there have been several troublesome mishaps.' These 'mishaps' are not specified; neither does Pappworth need to add any comments of his own to this admission. He noted that there had even been occasions in the published records when controversial 'details and complications' had been cut.

140

The original edition of *Human Guinea Pigs* concluded with words contributed by Sir Robert Hutchison to the *BMJ* in 1953: 'From inability to let well alone, from too much zeal for the new, and contempt for what is old; from putting knowledge before wisdom, science before art, cleverness before common sense; from treating patients as cases; and from making "the cure" of the disease more grievous than the endurance of the same, Good Lord deliver us.' One can see why, in both its sentiments and its rhetoric, this passage would have appealed to Maurice Pappworth. Once again, he let the words speak for themselves.

Reason and passion: the fuel for reform

A chief criticism of *Human Guinea Pigs* was that Pappworth used excessively graphic, even alarmist language – although in his review of the book for the *New Statesman* on 26 May 1967, the writer Arthur Koestler declared that 'Pappworth avoids emotionalism, utters his *j'accuse* in dry restrained tones.' Certainly his choice of vocabulary in describing research practices and attitudes he abhorred was part of his overall strategy. On one point he must, however, be defended from the start: he did go to considerable lengths to clarify medical terms for the lay reader. Words from 'clinical' to 'catheter,' from 'cannula' to 'cyanosed' are explained in footnotes at the bottom of the page. Reading *Human Guinea Pigs*, especially when doctors are quoted, enables the lay person to absorb, and after a while instinctively understand, much medical jargon. This links naturally with Pappworth's skills as a teacher.

As Helen Bamber recalled in her interview with Allan Gaw, Pappworth was always explaining. He engages with the reader, crediting him with the intelligence to reach his own judgments. He is sparing in his use of the rhetorical question, though occasionally we come across a sentence such as 'What experimenter… would submit his own child… wife… parent… to…?' He is impatient of non-sequiturs and alert to any lack of clarity. When considering, for instance, whether a procedure he describes is of benefit to the patient or purely experimental, Pappworth identifies 'ambiguity'. Scouring the medical journals for reports on research, Pappworth swooped on words he suspected to be deliberately ambiguous: 'What do the experimenters mean by the epithets "seldom", "reasonable" and "modest"?'

But there can be no doubt that, partly from the passion that marked the man and his attitudes, partly to achieve maximum impact, Pappworth used some high-flown vocabulary – not only to shock but also to amuse, in a kind of alliance with the reader. One of his postgraduate students was 'inveigled'; it is 'deplorable' that some doctors regard their patients as 'possessions'; we have become 'blinded by the razzle-dazzle of modern science'; research papers 'now constitute the royal road to getting on in the medical world'. Some of the strong language originates from other doctors. For example, he quotes Beecher on claims for the good of society being merely a 'cloak' for 'outrageous acts' and Whitehorn on physicians' 'phony attitude of omniscience'.

Pappworth loved to talk. He was a spell-binding lecturer, who loved reading and using words. By its very nature, *Human Guinea Pigs* offered the platform for his rhetorical flourishes. The following trio of sentences provide a good example of his skills in exploiting vocabulary and syntax to best effect: 'Undoubtedly no code can ever be a substitute for the moral integrity of any individual investigator. No code will curb the unscrupulous. No appeal to the conscience will be effective with anybody who lacks a conscience.'

In the special supplement to the Pelican edition of *Human Guinea Pigs*, Pappworth refers to Koestler's review, defending himself against those who criticised the way he wrote in the 1967 book. 'Some doctors have claimed that my language is too dramatic and emotive, and they cite in evidence my frequent use of terms such as "wide-bore needle" and "tightly fitting face mask and nose clip," and my giving the exact length of cardiac catheters used. But these are actual quotations from the published articles written by the experimenters themselves; I invented none of them.' More valid, perhaps, was the criticism levelled at Pappworth's choice of an emotive word such as 'stabbing' when 'inserting' might have been used instead. A careful reading of the book shows that such instances are not particularly common – though they were certainly a mainstay of the line chosen by some reviewers, especially those in medical journals.

It was felt that overblown language brought the medical profession into disrepute. This rather missed the point, of course. A profession stands or falls on its perceived and proven behaviour, not on the language its critics choose to employ. To the fury of the establishment, Pappworth took no hostages. *Human Guinea Pigs* is indeed, as Dr James Le Fanu describes it, 'an incredibly pugnacious book. You really admire him for not pulling his punches.' In his lectures at medical schools, as in his book, Pappworth would point the finger at professors at the very institutions in which he spoke. In Le Fanu's view, this, and the *ad hominem* accusations in *Human Guinea Pigs*, contain an element of revenge, of 'up yours'. As his former student Dr Barry Hoffbrand succinctly observes:

'*Human Guinea Pigs* was a *consequence* of Pappworth's and the medical profession's mutual attitude to each other.'

Human Guinea Pigs brought Pappworth both friends and enemies, as he knew it would, and enunciated some of his most strongly held views on medical practice and medical education. He was deeply troubled by the attitude of some researchers who, eager to push forward the frontiers of knowledge, were tempted into 'behaviour that many lay and medical people would regard as inhumane and at odds with their true calling'. To identify what he saw as a doctor's 'true calling' is to tell us much about Pappworth's professional ideals. He deplored the emphasis on research, rather than care of patients, as the surest way to career success, the urge to publish having become a 'maniacal impulse'. 'This is the case at some of the highest sources of medical teaching and, as a result, many of the most intelligent young doctors may spend several years after qualification right away from patients and engrossed in back-room techniques.' Early in *Human Guinea Pigs* Pappworth observes, 'The degree to which anti-humanism dominates modern medicine can be judged by the significant fact that, in most medical reports of patients having been submitted to experimentation, the patients themselves are collectively described as "the material".'

The term 'bedside manner' may nowadays sound absurdly quaint and old-fashioned, but it is what Pappworth believed in. As Helen Bamber put it: 'There was a purity that he had in terms of medicine... The patient came first and the patient was to be listened to.' Still in the early pages of *Human Guinea Pigs*, he complained that doctors obsessed with developing new scientific and technical advances 'have never developed the art of taking patients' histories properly. They have come to despise ordinary clinical examination of patients by the established means of using their eyes and hands and... simple instruments.' Anyone who has been thoroughly examined by a doctor prepared to take time and trouble, for whom at that moment you are apparently the most important person in the world, will know what Pappworth meant.

As shown in the cases he chose to expose, Pappworth, as a doctor and as an individual who had himself felt attacked and alone, believed in standing up for the weak. 'Every patient who becomes an experimental subject... is entitled to special consideration simply by virtue of the fact that, being a patient, he or she is a sick person. The same applies, I think, to a woman who is pregnant, to a mental defective or someone who is mentally ill, to a man in prison, to an old person, and to anyone whose disease is fatal, progressive and incurable (in other words, who is dying). It also applies to a volunteer who... is in a dependent relationship to the doctors conducting the experiment.' Infants and children he swiftly gathers under his protective wing. Pappworth did not become a father until he was forty-four, but he always showed a particular fondness for young children, even buying sweets for small strangers he encountered in shops – a habit from which he would not emerge unscathed nowadays. He describes those with mental illness as 'these unfortunate people', declaring himself 'shocked by students of my own who would favour the mass killing of psychotics'. 'At what point on the road to "elimination",' he asks (quoting the words of Nobel Prize-winning surgeon Alexis Carrel, uttered in 1939) 'do we call a halt?'

Dr Desmond Lawrence, in an interview with Charlie Gibbs, described Pappworth as 'the most combative man I have ever met'. Perhaps such a dubious distinction is inevitable in a whistle-blower, for he is certain he has found the most unassailable weapons: the weapons of proof. Allan Gaw, a confessed admirer, grants that Pappworth 'may be labelled as either a selfless champion or a bitter muckraker, wreaking revenge on a medical community that rejected him.' He was without doubt an angry man but, in the words of Helen Bamber, who worked so closely with him, 'not angry in a flamboyant way – in a quiet way feeling the pain and the anger. He felt very keenly.' Interestingly, she also believed that, once he had written the book, 'he didn't really want to see the material again... He'd got it down, and I think it was as much as he could do. It was a terribly painful thing for him to do.'

Plaudits and outrage: media and medical responses

So the monster-baby unleashed. How did the world respond? As with any medical story, the national press showed great interest. The Pappworths were not ex-directory, and once reviews started to appear, the phone was very busy, with members of the public ringing in to tell the whistle-blower about their experiences. I remember taking a number of calls and handing them over to my father. He stayed very calm, and didn't on the whole seem interested in adding their tales to a dossier for future editions of the book.

One of the earliest reviews to appear was written by Donald Trelford in *The Observer* on 14 May. In it he predicted that it was 'likely to lead to fresh demands for control of hospital experiments'. The BBC Magazine, *The Listener*, included a review by Bernard Williams in the middle of June, which called *Human Guinea Pigs* a 'disturbing book' and 'not altogether an easy book to read. A good part of it consists of a formidable, but inevitably rather repetitious, assemblage of cases from the medical literature; and some of the material... is likely to make the unhardened non-medical reader feel pretty ill.' Williams advises 'a certain amount of skipping to avoid boredom or queasiness,' but maintains that 'the general upshot of the evidence should not be ignored.'

One of the most interesting lay reviews appeared in the *New Statesman*, on 26 May. Penned by Arthur Koestler, and sub-titled 'Dr Moreau's Modern Islands', it was – as one might expect from the independent-minded journalist, novelist and campaigner – thoughtful, original, and neither wholly for or against. 'Faith in the omniscience of the medical man is an essential element in all healing and he who shatters that faith assumes a responsibility towards the patient comparable to the physician's,' the writer declares. 'A semi-educated person superficially browsing through the more lurid pages of Dr Pappworth's book, might easily jump to the conclusion that to go to a hospital for a minor operation is equivalent to being lured to the islands of Dr Moreau and vivisected by a team of researchers with steely eyes above white masks.'

He continues that "When the macabre aura surrounding these experiments is dispelled and emotionalism bred by ignorance discounted, there remains a hard core of cases in Dr Pappworth's list where his criticisms seem to be fully justified. This applies particularly to some experiments carried out on children, on pregnant women, mental defectives, on patients before and after an operation, and on those with incurable diseases; and to a lesser extent on prisoner volunteers.'

But when Pappworth claims that 'the ethical problems arising from human experimentation have become one of the cardinal issues of our time,' Koestler criticises this as 'one of the few overstatements in his book,' adding that 'it is a monumental one'. Koestler believed that 'the horrors' of experimentation on human beings described by Pappworth may be 'on the wane'. He concludes, '*Human Guinea Pigs* is a book to be pondered by the profession. There is less point in recommending it to the general public – which has other "cardinal issues" to worry about.'

It was the *Daily Express* that kicked off the national press coverage on 9 May, with a brief news report by James Wilkinson under the headline 'What *are* your chances of being a hospital guinea pig?' The *Daily Mail* followed swiftly on 15 May, shortly before publication: 'The Harley Street specialist, consultant physician Dr Maurice Pappworth, 57, alleges that children, pregnant women, mental defectives and old people were being used in National Health hospitals as "guinea pigs" without consent... He claims that recovery was sometimes delayed in the interests of medical research, and likens some of the experiments to research carried out at the Nazi concentration camps during the war.'

News articles appeared in *The Times* on 18 and 20 May, on the same dates in *The Guardian*, and a press conference was organised to coincide with publication. In an article which conceded that the tone of Pappworth's writing was 'emotional' and therefore 'enough to let the medical profession pooh-pooh his arguments', Ann Shearer of The Guardian quoted a doctor whose view, voiced at the press conference, damningly let slip the prevalent attitude of the medical establishment: 'it was "useless to explain to a charwoman what was going to be done because she could not possibly understand."' Pappworth's MRCP students revelled in the publicity their teacher was attracting – though as one later remarked in the *BMJ*, 'Ironically he himself became an integral part of the machinery he despised and soon found fame... on his way to international "celebrity" status.' This may be something of an exaggeration, but usefully reminds us that Pappworth wrote *Human Guinea Pigs* neither for money or fame. The truth, as he saw it, had to be spoken, and it was his privilege or his nemesis to be the one to do it.

One unintended consequence of the publication of *Human Guinea Pigs*, and the press interest it garnered, was its effect on Maurice Pappworth's brother Sidney. The rent in their relationship caused by disagreement over their father's final illness had not been repaired, and Maurice did not bother to tell his brother about the forthcoming book. Sidney's younger daughter Rachel records that at least one of the cases cited named a doctor who worked at the same hospital as her father. All the local newspapers pointed out that Maurice Pappworth's brother was Senior Consultant and Head of Accident and Emergency at the very hospital where one of the cases described had occurred. 'This caused my father a lot of problems, as the implication was that he must have provided [Maurice] with the information that he used in his book.' Both Sidney's daughters emphasise, however, that the principles informing *Human Guinea Pigs* – with the needs of the patient placed above all else – were ones which both their doctor parents wholeheartedly endorsed.

For *The Economist,* in a review on 20 May, 'On the evidence scrupulously documented in this book, some practitioners of experimental medicine are wolves in white coats and are prepared to do hair-raising things to people submitted to a hospital's care.' The reviewer goes on to observe that Pappworth 'is out to give a much-needed shock and will not be popular in medical high places; but he is right to insist that scientific enthusiasm should be tempered by humanity and prudence, and that the patient's interests should at all times be paramount.'

Local newspapers also took an interest – for example the *Hampstead and Highgate Express*, home to both Maurice Pappworth and the Royal Free Hospital, which came in for some criticism. Under the headline 'No "guinea pigs" at Royal Free,' the reporter informed readers that the hospital's administrator, Gordon Heppell, 'gave an assurance this week that experiments are not carried out on patients without their consent and without their being told of what is involved'. At the top of the article, Pappworth's handwritten note remarks, 'Obviously not read book which has plentiful named references to Royal Free.'

On the other side of the Atlantic, where an American edition was in preparation, a review in the *New York Times* on 14 July by Dr Michael Halberstam stated that Pappworth documented 'convincingly... an excessive trust in scientific medicine and our own profession in particular'. Halberstam referred to the 'corruption' which Pappworth 'clearly reveals'. In *Human Guinea Pigs*, Pappworth worked 'relentlessly' to make his case, and was, the American doctor assured us, 'no fanatic.' Too often, 'research physicians lose sight of the particular patient... No physician who reads this book will ever make that mistake again and we shall all be the better for it.'

Responses to the book in medical journals were often hostile – just as Pappworth expected. The anonymous 'Hamster' of *Hospital Medicine* described it as 'an irresponsible piece of work, which will sadden, rather than infuriate the profession. Nothing or no-one appears to be sacred to him, and however genuine his motives in writing the book, it may well be that he defeats his own purpose.... The fact that so many lives are saved by the struggles of doctors and scientists, should be enough to put Dr Pappworth's dogma into its proper place – the waste chute.' There was lively debate, including a letter from Pappworth defending his position, in the correspondence section of *Hospital Medicine*. Pappworth was also condemned in the *Medical Tribune* on 25 May: he had 'made a terrible error and has wronged many honest men by comparing research done in British hospitals to the Nazi experiments on human beings in concentration camps of the last war... It is a great pity that he has used such hideous comparisons in trying to make his case.' This was to be a theme picked up later in Parliamentary discussions on the book and its call for legislation.

On the same date, possibly the most damning professional review of *Human Guinea Pigs* was penned by Dr Christopher Booth for the *International Medical*

Tribune of Great Britain. It later emerged that Booth was among those who strenuously opposed Pappworth's election to a Fellowship of the Royal College of Physicians, and there is without doubt an element of personal vindictiveness in his review. Booth was not an impartial commentator, being at the time a recently-appointed professor and director of medicine at the Hammersmith Hospital: one of Pappworth's chief targets. He was an influential doctor, who was knighted in 1983 and went on to become president of the BMA: in other words, the classic establishment figure from whom the outsider Pappworth felt alienated.

Picking up on exactly the phrase that Arthur Koestler was to query, Booth quotes Pappworth's statement that 'the ethical problems involved in medical research have become one of the cardinal issues of our time'. Yet, Booth tells us, 'it is palpably untrue to claim... that the majority of doctors are either genuinely ignorant of the immensity and complexity of the problem, or wish purposely to ignore the whole matter by sweeping it under the carpet... His book treats the serious subject of the involvement of human beings in research without sufficient understanding, personal experience, or knowledge. His work can only have the effect of alarming those whom doctors seek to relieve of diseases which cripple and kill them... Which does most harm? Suspicion or confidence?'

Booth refers to 'one of Dr Pappworth's recent alarms' on the BBC radio programme *The World at One*, after which 'two of my patients, on whom the effects of a standard treatment for asthma were being carefully measured by simple tests, refused to continue the treatment because they thought they were being experimented on.' He goes on to deplore 'how easily a lay-interviewer may be misled by an obsessional doctor with a special bone to pick with his colleagues'. Booth concludes that Pappworth 'is to be condemned for his continued public attacks on his professional colleagues who, by their research, are doing all they can to improve the treatment they give to sick people who come to them for help'.

Booth seems to have been rattled by the volume of media coverage Pappworth was receiving. And it was coverage that Pappworth desired. He took Booth's review as a salvo to which he should return fire in a letter. 'Professor Booth is as evasive as other of his colleagues... He should have stated that he is on the staff of Hammersmith Hospital and a biased reviewer. Will he please give unequivocal answers to the following questions concerning references to his hospital made in my book: 1) Did the experiments, which I describe, take place? 2) Were they published? This in itself indicates a certain pride in what was done. 3) Are there any factual errors in my summaries...?' So he continues, determined to make the point that the gruesome experiments undertaken at the Hammersmith really did take place and that the researchers were pleased with their work. He asks if Booth advocates 'obedience to the maxim *primum non nocere*' [above all, do no harm] and, in response to Booth's claim that 'Many schools of medicine have set up research committees to examine and appraise all clinical research projects,' points out that 'he fails to mention that this is one of the recommendations advised by me'.

On 6 June *World Medicine* ran a 'Controversy' feature, including photos of both Pappworth and his old television adversary Dr Charles Fletcher – another key member of the Hammersmith team. As had become the norm, he accused the author of *Human Guinea Pigs* of using 'highly dramatic terms' when describing experiments and dismissed the legal code proposed in the book as 'quite impracticable'. Pappworth may have felt hemmed in by his adversaries, but he himself courted exposure on the battlefield. And he was not without his supporters. Many doctors were prepared to express their agreement only privately, but it is interesting to note that a member of the public, one C. Fettes, wrote to the editor of *Medical News* at the end of June asking if 'a mere layman' could be allowed to comment on Pappworth's book. The correspondent notes that there has been, in doctors' reactions to *Human Guinea Pigs*, a tendency to 'naively assume that no member of the medical profession would ever dream of putting his own advancement before the welfare of his fellow men. Thus your only response to Dr Pappworth's laudable attempt to redeem the reputation of your profession by purging it of unscrupulous elements is to talk of the many lives "saved by the struggles of doctors and scientists": would you equally suggest that corrupt policemen should not be arrested because the majority of their colleagues are honest and hard-working?'

The debate was still rumbling four years later, when Dr John McRae – a former student of Pappworth's, and a family friend – named to *The Times* four London teaching hospitals in which, he alleged, unjustified experiments were being conducted. He claimed that patients of his had been experimented on at the Westminster Children's, the Charing Cross, St Thomas's and University College. The article concluded: 'Acting on recommendation by a committee of the Royal College of Physicians, almost all teaching hospitals and many district hospitals have set up ethical committees.' The wheels were well and truly turning now. But it was a hard road, and the more stubbornly he trod, the more enemies Pappworth seemed to be marking – including those who had once been friends.

On 2 September 1972, Pappworth received a reply written on behalf of Lord [Henry] Cohen of Birkenhead, President of the General Medical Council, regarding the necessary procedures if a complaint was to be brought against doctors considered 'guilty of serious professional misconduct'. The letter is an attempt to fob off the dogged Dr Pappworth. What is most interesting, however, is that Lord Cohen, who from 1934 held the Chair of Medicine at the University of Liverpool and had been Pappworth's revered teacher, chose not to answer the letter himself. Instead, he arranged for his registrar to write to his former student.

Cohen had become part of the medical establishment. As a result, it would seem that both he and Pappworth now saw each other from opposite sides of a field they had once shared. In a letter to *World Medicine*, Pappworth openly attacked his former teacher and friend: 'Why has not Lord Cohen publicly condemned the use of hospital patients for hazardous experiments without valid consent? He has claimed to me personally that he has read my book and thus has all the required evidence.'

Political procrastination

One anonymous reviewer described *Human Guinea Pigs* as a book 'written with a chip on the shoulder'. In a sense, however, any subconscious motivation in writing it was immaterial. Pappworth wanted to get something done. His chief hope was that response to his revelations would attract attention all the way to the top, and that his suggestions – notably with regard to the establishment of ethical committees – would be acted on by government. But the Labour government of the time, headed by Prime Minister Harold Wilson, did not seem to be interested. It may simply have been a question of civil servants at the Ministry of Health becoming increasingly obstinate in the face of Pappworth's campaign.

Events had started to unfold even before the publication of *Human Guinea Pigs*. A representative of the Patients' Association wrote to Minister of Health Kenneth Robinson in early May demanding an investigation: the Association had been tipped off about the allegations to be made. In the *Evening Standard* of 17 May, Helen Hodgson, Chair of the Patients' Association (who had appeared with Pappworth and Fletcher on *This Week* four years earlier), announced: 'The cases listed by Dr Pappworth seem to be perfectly cut and dried... Dr Pappworth's book is likely to cause a great deal of public alarm and concern.'

But in late May the minister refused the Patients' Association demand for an inquiry into the general question of experiments on patients. *The Times* claimed on 20 May that the confidence of the Ministry of Health had been 'shaken' after a letter backed by the association was sent in support of an inquiry. The following day, a letter to the *Observer* from K.G. Perona-Wright, of the Fountain and Carshalton Hospital Group, referred readers back to early December 1961. The then Minister of Health, Enoch Powell, had made a statement in the House of Commons concerning an experiment on children conducted in a number of hospitals, including Fountain and Carshalton, to test out a measles vaccination. These trials had been a target of Pappworth's criticism. Powell confirmed that the parents of these children had given their consent in writing. Immediately following this letter, the *Observer* printed one from the indomitable Helen Hodgson, who claimed that 'Patients in hospital are under considerable pressure to accept whatever is suggested to them, as they cannot assess the risks involved.'

Joyce Butler, the Labour MP for Wood Green, took up the cause, endorsing the Patients' Association in asking the Minister to appoint a committee of inquiry. Kenneth Robinson's response was an uncompromising 'No'. As he explains, 'Comprehensive guidance to doctors was given in this matter by the Medical Research Council in its reports for 1962-3 and in September 1964... If my honourable friend cares to draw my attention to any subsequent specific case in which there is *prima facie* evidence that the guidance has not been followed by hospital doctors in England and Wales, I shall be glad to look into it.' So the minister was, in a somewhat offhand manner, placing responsibility for further investigations in the court of Mrs Butler and the Patients' Association. And, of course, of Maurice Pappworth.

'The official attitude,' insisted the Ministry of Health, 'is that the Minister does not give instructions to doctors on matters of professional conduct.' A spokesman declared that the disciplinary body for doctors was the General Medical Council, adding 'There is no specialist law relating to this question, but patients are protected by the general laws relating to assault and damages.' So far as the government was concerned, the medical profession was policing itself and there was no need for further legislation to protect the interests of patients.

Nearly five years later, in January 1972, Joyce Butler was given leave to introduce the Rights of Patients Bill. It aimed to clarify the rights of patients to privacy when receiving hospital treatment under the NHS, and also with regard to medical experiments on human beings. *The Times* reported that although it was not possible to 'legislate for human behaviour,' the patient's right to 'refuse to be used as teaching material and the duty of hospitals to inform them of that right' could be written into law. 'Because of the public concern aroused by reports of human guinea pigs in hospitals,' *The Times* noted, Mrs Butler had 'included reference to it in the Bill. Hospitals had been asked to establish committees and the Department of Social Security was making inquiries as to how many hospitals had done this.' After a dispiriting start, progress was eventually made in the campaign for ethical committees. It was a struggle, not least because, as one former Pappworth student remarked to me, 'Politicians don't like doctors; doctors don't like politicians.' Nothing much has changed there.

Julian Snow, Parliamentary Secretary to the Ministry of Health, spoke in the Commons in June about *Human Guinea Pigs* in response to continuing demands for an inquiry. He declared that 'my interest in this book lapsed when I saw that Dr Pappworth was equating British doctors with Nazi concentration camp doctors.' The response by columnist 'Peter Simple' (pen-name of Michael Wharton) in the *Daily Telegraph* on 21 June, in a piece entitled 'Unfortunate Lapse', was to ask, 'What sort of argument is that? If Dr Pappworth's book really does "equate British doctors with Nazi concentration camp doctors," shouldn't Mr Snow's interest, far from lapsing, have been greatly intensified? The Ministry of Health is supposed to be concerned with medical practice, not with the political history of the Second World War and with possible affronts to British patriotic feeling. Nobody imagines that British doctors are experimenting on patients without their consent for precisely the same reasons as Nazi concentration camp doctors once did. What chiefly matters now is: are they doing so at all, and if so, what is the Ministry of Health going to do about it?'

In a House of Lords debate on 25 January 1973, on a government bill about NHS reorganisation, Lord Beaumont proposed an amendment to make medical ethical committees a statutory obligation for all NHS hospitals in which studies on patients were being done, stating that at least a quarter of the committee's members should not be doctors, para-medical workers, or anybody else employed in the NHS. The amendment was seconded by Lord Strabolgi, who pointed out that demands for an inquiry into alleged unethical clinical experiments had been turned down on three separate occasions. It was Lord Platt, at the time President of the Royal College of Physicians, who opposed the amendment, on the grounds that it was it was impossible to define the term 'experiment'. Meanwhile Lord Brock, President of the Royal College of Surgeons, maintained that 'The provision of these ethical committees is not a suitable subject for legislation. We should leave things as they are and trust in the good sense and responsibility of the doctors.' His lordship had, perhaps deliberately, missed the point of Pappworth's argument.

Towards the end of his 1990 article '*Human Guinea Pigs* – A History', Pappworth, more in anger than in sorrow, claims that 'There is strong evidence that few doctors have read my book.' Apparently, he asked the audience of over one hundred staff to whom he was lecturing at the Hammersmith Hospital how many of them had read *Human Guinea Pigs*, and 'only two raised a hand'. When, early in his career, Professor Robert Winston was working at the Hammersmith as a researcher, he noted how his senior colleagues 'furiously condemned Pappworth' for the publication of *Human Guinea Pigs*. In *Bad Ideas* (2010), however, he claimed that within months of the book's appearance the Hammersmith set up 'excellent ethical committees to ensure good clinical conduct and proper patient consent for all researchers.'

To the end Pappworth maintained that his methods had been the only effective ones. He contrasted these with the more cautious line adopted by Henry Beecher. The latter had claimed that his decision not to name names in his 1964 article in the *New England Journal of Medicine* was taken on legal grounds, as the investigators might have found themselves liable to criminal proceedings. 'I believe that giving names and references has, at least in small measure, acted as a deterrent.' He also pointed out that insurance companies in Australia refused to give cover to doctors who engaged in research on patients unless their work had been agreed by an ethical committee. Of course Pappworth wished to seize on any positive outcome of his book, but there remained a sense of disappointment. The ethical committees that finally emerged had many shortcomings, as recognised in a 1990 editorial in the *BMJ*: that their establishment was not mandatory and they had no legal status continued to haunt the author of *Human Guinea Pigs*.

Chapter Seven

The patient's champion, the doctor's conscience: a career in controversy

'My opinion remains that those who dirty the linen and not those who wash it should be criticised. Some do not wash dirty linen in public or in private and the dirt is merely left to accumulate until it stinks.'

(Maurice Pappworth, from an article in the British Medical Journal in 1990)

Ethical committees: an overdue birth

Fifty years after the publication of *Human Guinea Pigs*, we have to ask how much the book actually achieved. It certainly made doctors and patients sit up and take notice. The widespread press interest precipitated this – a further red rag to powerful medical professionals, who generally frowned upon contact with the media. It is probably fair to argue that *Human Guinea Pigs* speeded up what was already being implemented with dragging heels. Ethical committees were established after a slow start, for they were all about controlling doctors, who did not like being controlled. The committees which Pappworth had advocated came into being in hospitals throughout Britain twenty years behind the setting up of ethical review boards in the United States.

Interestingly, in the autobiographical tape Pappworth made, he says very little about *Human Guinea Pigs*. He barely touches on the struggles before and after its publication. Instead, he offers us just three sentences. 'Other important aspects of my career were the publication of three successful books. First, *Human Guinea Pigs* which was published by Routledge and also as a Penguin, and translated into Italian and German. This caused a great controversy at the time and was in fact the reason for the establishment of ethical committees in the United Kingdom.'

This last point shows Pappworth was confident that he could claim responsibility for the committees. It is made again in an article he wrote for *World Medicine* in 1978 on the subject of research ethical committees: 'My own first questioning of the ethics and even legality of some research was in 1960, and in that same year I appeared on several radio and TV programmes discussing the problem.' Looking back, nearly twenty years later, when the media had become more ubiquitous and sophisticated, he recognised the importance of setting up a high profile. He notes in the same article that the Royal College of Physicians had already started looking into the establishment of ethical committees before the book was published – the implication being that the College anticipated the commotion which *Human Guinea Pigs* would inspire, and believed it needed to be seen to be doing something.

In 1967, the RCP published its *Report of the Committee on the Supervision of the Ethics of Clinical Investigations in Institutions*. This recommended that in medical institutions where clinical research is carried out, all projects should be approved by a group of doctors including those experienced in clinical investigation. It declared that the relevant authority had a duty to 'ensure that all clinical investigations carried out within its hospital or institution are ethical and conducted with the optimum technical skill and precautions for safety'. As Charlie Gibbs notes, 'This marked the start of a process in the implementation of ethics committees that would eventually oversee the ethical liability of experiments carried out within all NHS hospitals.' Writing on 30 April to Professor Desmond Laurence of University College Hospital, a member of the 1967 RCP committee, to thank him for sending a pre-publication copy, Pappworth could not resist adding a touch of salt: 'What intrigues me most is why the RCP made their recommendations in 1967, as though medical research had suddenly become a new activity?'

Notwithstanding his gratitude to Laurence for giving him a sneak preview of the RCP report, Pappworth, in a September 1967 letter to the *BMJ*, dismissed it as a 'white-washing, worthless document, purposely vague'. He was disappointed that the RCP report failed to recommend his proposal that ethical committees should include lay members of the public.

However, the work of the Royal College did not stop with its 1967 Report. The College's Annals show that in April 1973 – the year in which the 1967 working party's report was made public – an important meeting took place. The ten-strong Committee on the Supervision of the Ethics of Clinical Research Investigations in Institutions, chaired by Dr D.A. Clarke and observed by a medical representative from the Department of Health and Social Security, was still catching the fall-out of *Human Guinea Pigs*. This committee aimed to provide more detailed recommendations on the 'composition and scope' of ethical committees 'as requested by the Chief Medical Officer'. Here, essentially, was an admission of the inadequacies of the College's report six years earlier: a damage-limitation exercise was necessary. 'The object of ethical committees,' according to the minutes, 'is to safeguard patients, healthy volunteers and the reputation of the profession and its institutions in matters of clinical research investigation.'

The 1973 minutes recommend that, in order to 'function efficiently' ethical committees should be small, and 'they must not be so constituted as to cause an unreasonable hindrance to the advancement of medical knowledge'. In other words, there must be plenty of practising doctors represented. These medical professionals should be 'experienced clinicians with a knowledge of clinical research investigation'. In addition, there should be a lay member. The recommendations go on to define a lay person as 'an individual who is not associated with the profession in any paramedical activity, i.e. a biochemist or a psychologist would not be considered as a layman for this purpose.' Clearly there was no place on an ethical committee for nurses, who did not fall into the 'clinician' category, but would have been loosely considered to belong to the 'paramedical' class. Specialists from outside the committee would, it was recognised, have to be called in sometimes to testify. The minutes of the 1973 committee meeting indicate that the composition of ethical committees was a sensitive topic, judging by views expressed in the College's Survey Report of 1971. It was estimated that about one-fifth of all ethical committees included lay members and 'it may be that we should recommend general extension of this practice'. This would have been a move welcomed by Pappworth, who was a strong advocate of the contribution to be made on ethical questions by lay people, notably lawyers and theologians.

Tellingly, the committee recommended that, although research intended to benefit the patient should normally be accompanied by the subject's full and informed consent, there were also 'circumstances in which it is inappropriate or even inhumane to explain the details and seek consent'. These evidently gruesome procedures were just such as those described in *Human Guinea Pigs*. The 1973 recommendations leave it to individual ethical committees to examine such cases 'with particular care'. This report hedges its bets on research carried out on children and 'mentally handicapped' adults, claiming that these 'may be permissible', but acknowledging that, although the parent or guardian's permission should be recorded, 'legally no-one has the right to give consent for experiments to be carried out on another person'. It quotes the Medical Research Council's statement regarding untested therapies or procedures: 'the relationship is essentially between doctor and patient'. But it was precisely to protect patients from the occasional unscrupulous doctor that ethical committees were formed. There is an admission that it is 'both considerate and prudent' to obtain a patient's agreement. Pappworth would have groaned at such bromide adjectives. To him, and to many like-minded people, ensuring that the patient gives informed consent is vital, and the imperative moral starting-point for any investigation.

The 1973 committee must have recognised that not all doctors can be relied upon to take a compassionate and disinterested view on the hazards to which they may be submitting their patients. For one important recommendation, appearing towards the end of the minutes, wonders 'whether there might be advantage in some central body, perhaps within the College, to which local committees could turn for advice in difficult cases and which could issue guidance illustrated by accounts of actual cases'. The committee was thinking things through carefully: its suggestions and recommendations on the composition and monitoring of ethical committees, its focus on the question of consent, and the suggestion that a guiding body might be set up to advise on ethical matters, all indicate that Pappworth's book and the subsequent controversy was still having an effect.

But did the College have a self-interested motive? Why did it assemble this committee when, as Pappworth himself suggested, the report on ethical supervision brought out in 1967 was, essentially, a publicity exercise before the can of worms opened that summer with the publication of *Human Guinea Pigs*? The minutes reveal the College's motivation through the words of the 1973 committee chairman, Dr Clarke, who refers to the 'background of heavy pressure on our Ministers to institute an enquiry into allegations of unethical practices in experimentation made against certain teaching hospitals'.

Not once is Maurice Pappworth and his whistle-blowing book named. The chairman continues that 'we wished to follow up the Royal College of Physicians' survey of hospital authorities' progress in establishing ethical committees with an enquiry of our own. The enquiry showed, he claims, that all teaching hospital authorities, and more than three-quarters of others where clinical research was undertaken, had established ethical committees, or used another committee – normally the medical advisory committee – to consider ethical issues pertaining to their research. It had clearly been recognised that, while ethical committees or their equivalent were now mandatory, these still required detailed oversight.

Political uneasiness is also suggested by Clarke's reference to the question asked in the House of Commons on the subject in January 1972. The Parliamentary Secretary's response had been to offer talks between the Department of Health and 'the professional bodies concerned'. Here was a matter that the medical profession needed to be seen to confront. Some eminent doctors certainly wished to continue the pressure. Pappworth was pleased to receive a supportive letter from Sir Francis Avery Jones, a physician at the Central Middlesex Hospital and a widely respected medical figure, which he quotes in his 1990 article for the BMJ on *Human Guinea Pigs*. Avery Jones also wrote to the General Medical Council in March 1974 expressing concern that still not enough was being done to rectify the abuses catalogued in the book. But many continued to find Pappworth, the small, stubborn Scouser, over-emotional and lacking in objectivity. This becomes a problem in trying to assess the impact of *Human Guinea Pigs*. *Did* this unrelenting pursuer of his cause alienate too many people, meaning that the book's influence was more of an *indirect* one, rather than a personal triumph?

In 1984, the Royal College of Physicians issued new guidelines, and in 1985 a committee of twenty-two was set up to consider them. Its report, published in January 1990, was described at the end of that year by Pappworth in his *BMJ* article as 'excellent'. Margaret Turner-Warwick, then President of the Royal College of Physicians, summarised the history of this process, which spanned twenty-three years: 'In 1967 the RCP recommended that research involving patients and normal subjects should undergo ethical review. This led to the establishment of local Research Ethics Committees. The College feels that it has now become necessary to review and update the Guidelines. They deliberately refrained from dictating a right solution.'

Celebrity – and ostracism

Ultimately, Pappworth stands firmly in the ranks of those who are prepared to put their careers on the line for the sake of the truth. In naming names, he succeeded, as he himself later noted, in establishing a kind of deterrent. 'The great thing about [Pappworth],' remarked Desmond Laurence in an interview with Charlie Gibbs, 'was that he named names.' Allan Gaw concludes in his 2009 *BMJ* article, 'Finding Maurice Pappworth', that *Human Guinea Pigs* 'is now regarded as a major milestone on the journey towards the modern system of research ethics committee review'.

In Gibbs' view, the book 'went a long way to creating the will and political climate' that led to those committees, 'even though Pappworth himself was ostracised by most of the medical community'. Again, the word 'whistle-blower' is used to describe him. 'I think he did have an impact,' declared Pappworth's collaborator Helen Bamber in her interview with Gaw. 'He did make change.' In Bamber's work for the Medical Foundation for the Care of Victims of Torture, which she set up in 1985, Pappworth's influence is evident.

In June 1968, a year after the publication of *Human Guinea Pigs*, *World Medicine* ran a piece covering a recent discussion at the Royal Society of Medicine in which Pappworth was joined by Professor John Butterfield, Professor of Medicine at Guy's Hospital, and the writer and broadcaster Edgar Lustgarten. Characteristic quotations from Pappworth's opening salvo include a reference to 'the current craze for so-called routine investigations' and the 'phoney omniscience' presented to their patients by too many doctors. In another favourite phrase picked up by the *World Medicine* reporter, Pappworth declared that people could not be made 'martyrs for society'. Writing to me forty-eight years after the publication of this article, a former President of the Royal College of Physicians declared: 'How right [Pappworth] was, and how wrong was commonly accepted practice.' The rights of the individual, as against the needs of society, are today as hot a topic as ever.

Professor Butterfield avoided a direct confrontation with Pappworth but pointed out that rapid changes in the human environment meant that research in as-yet unexamined areas needed to be undertaken. He agreed the profession had to ensure that experimental medicine did not become the vehicle for an individual's ambition. Edgar Lustgarten, meanwhile, supported Pappworth's contention that ethical committees should include lay persons. Just as 'war was too important to be left to the generals,' so experimental ethics were 'too important to be left to the experts.' Certainly, by stressing the doctor's primary role as ensuring the welfare of individual patients, rather than the advancement of science, Lustgarten – a well-respected legal commentator – showed himself a Pappworth ally. He emphasised that the sanctity of the individual must at all times be maintained. In true Lustgarten style, he drew an analogy between Burke and Hare, who in 19th-century Edinburgh defiled the dead by robbing graves of corpses for medical experiments, and the doctors who carry out research on their patients and therefore defile the living.

A year later, in 1969, a Norwegian medical journal published an interview (in English) with Pappworth after he had delivered a university lecture in Norway. When asked why he wrote the book, Pappworth claimed 'I thought I had a contribution to make.' He was aware that many fellow professionals agreed with his concerns but were not prepared to speak out. 'I found... that these things will not stop until doctors are prepared, as I am, to come out into the open and name names and say that doctor X is one who is guilty of doing these things... I know for a fact since I published my book there has been a great slowing down on such experiments. On the other hand, a lot more secret work is going on.' He pointed out that in England there had been not a single legal action against any doctor on the grounds that he experimented on a patient without valid consent. 'If a person knows that, he is likely to take the risk.' Using the car analogy he so favoured, Pappworth pointed out that if no Norwegian motorist had ever been prosecuted for speeding, certain people would risk exceeding the limit.

As always, Pappworth underlined the key issues of valid consent, and the use of controls and volunteers. He enjoyed the company of lawyers, and would not have been exaggerating when he claimed that the many lawyers he had talked to considered doctors who undertook experimental work to be 'running a terrible risk'. He quoted a judge who observed that 'This field can be narrowed a good deal further by the law of trespass. It is actionable to interfere bodily with any other person without his consent, in the absence of clear therapeutic indications.' And he raised the critical question of 'do the ends justify the means?' He stated his conviction that 'putting science before public welfare and the obligation to the patient is wrong, and any claim to do so for the good of society should be regarded with extreme distaste and even alarm.'

A further interview with Pappworth appeared in September 1970 in *Hospital Times*. Dr Anthony Campbell's opening gambit was to ask Pappworth why so few doctors had read *Human Guinea Pigs*. 'Because they think they know all about it,' retorted Pappworth. 'Some have wanted to know whether or not they are mentioned in it. Some have said: "Thank God I've never done anything like that." I said: "But, you know, you're mentioned in my book."' He claimed that 'Nobody has denied that the experiments described did take place. The fact that they were published shows a pride in what was done.' He pointed out that nobody had sued him, but deeply regretted that those doctors who agreed with him were not prepared to speak out.

Towards the end of the interview, Pappworth states the controversial opinion he had already expressed on television: 'If by killing a few people you would thereby obtain a certain cure for cancer, would this be justifiable?... My answer is definitely no... It is again this notion of doing possible good to the greatest number.' Perhaps his stance arose partly from the Talmudic view that he who saves a single person saves the whole world. It is hard to think in terms of the suffering of one individual when set against a possible benefit to millions. But Pappworth was encouraging people to think about such important moral questions.

The debate continued sporadically but persistently throughout the years following the book's publication, and spread into other controversial areas of medicine. An article in the *Daily Telegraph* on 9 June 1970 covered a debate at the Cambridge Union, the motion being 'This House would not allow the State to make use of human organs once clinical death is established, other than those of people who have contracted into a central computerised register.' The motion was proposed by Dr M.H. Pappworth and opposed by Britain's leading liver transplant surgeon, Professor Roy Calne. The newspaper headline focused on Pappworth's claim that Calne was committing euthanasia, with reference to the Human Tissues Act. To Pappworth's accusation that 'All these transplant surgeons want is legalised euthanasia,' Calne responded that his opposite number had lowered the reputation of the medical profession, describing Pappworth as 'bigoted' and with no understanding of transplant surgery. The motion was carried by eighty-seven votes to twenty-one. Most striking, perhaps, were the questions Pappworth raised about the definition of death, and whether or not certain kinds of brain damage are irreversible. For they indicate that the moral issues in *Human Guinea Pigs* were part of a debate that will never end. The more medical science advances, the more that doctors and surgeons find that they are able to do, the more the ethical controversy continues.

March 1971 saw Pappworth writing to the *BMJ* to suggest the wording for a new Hippocratic Oath, the original having been removed from a doctor's graduation ritual in the 1950s. Unlike his letters of the previous two decades, this one was published. Three months later, *The Lancet* featured letters by both Pappworth and Henry Beecher of Harvard, the former on a recent case at Willowbank, an American hospital, where 'mentally defective' children were moved into a specialist liver unit and then submitted to a programme of liver trials.

Beecher, who had already written about this case in *The Lancet*, wrote a letter regretting the Medical Research Council's stonewalling when he sought clarification of their policy on parents and guardians giving consent on behalf of others. Toward the end of the year, on 17 November 1971, Pappworth's trenchant letter to the *Times* was published. Here he swooped on the Under Secretary for Health and Social Security, Michael Alison, whose answer to a question in the House of Commons showed he was scarcely aware of the stack of evidence of unethical experiments conducted in British hospitals brought to light in *Human Guinea Pigs*.

In the *Radio Times* in February 1972, Pappworth felt able to confirm that, since the publication of *Human Guinea Pigs*, the situation had 'improved slightly' with the creation of research ethical committees. But he insisted that unacceptable experiments continued at some teaching hospitals, with patients still in the dark about the exact nature of what was involved. Even in 1978, in an article for *World Medicine*, Pappworth was claiming that neither the General Medical Council in Britain nor the American medical associations were intervening 'meaningfully', being 'more concerned with medical etiquette than with ethics'. It is testament to Pappworth's unflagging adherence to his cause that, more than ten years after the publication of his book, he was still monitoring its practical outcomes. It was chiefly thanks to Pappworth – the right man at the right time – that a more compassionate and patient-centred approach started to infuse British medicine, particularly where scientific advances threatened to conflict with patients' needs. 'He was a rare being at that time,' mused Helen Bamber in 2011. 'I think medicine has changed a great deal.' One eminent doctor described Pappworth's book to me as one with 'global consequences'.

What was the impact on Pappworth himself of his courageous whistle-blowing? Although *Human Guinea Pigs* was commercially successful, he was ostracised by the medical profession. This is what happens to whistle-blowers, after all: the establishment closes ranks. As Allan Gaw strikingly puts in his article on the Pappworth/Beecher correspondence: 'Pappworth's whistleblowing strategy burst the eardrums of his profession.' As a result, he 'found himself vilified'. Normally, consultant physicians became Fellows of the Royal College of Physicians between ten and fifteen years after being awarded Membership. Today, Fellowship is automatically conferred fifteen years after the MRCP exam has been passed. But from Pappworth, the Fellowship was withheld for fifty-seven years.

There were other ramifications. Pappworth returned from a New Year holiday in the Far East with Jean in January 1968 to find a letter from Norman Franklin of Routledge enclosing a cutting from the *Evening Standard*: 'as you will see, the police are anxious to interview you'. The police, apparently, had been 'bothered by somebody who wanted to prosecute one of the people denounced in your book'. Michael Rubinstein had warned Franklin that an unsuccessful prosecution could result in a libel suit.

In the event, this incident came to nothing. But the fact that the *Evening Standard* chose to include Pappworth's police summons as a news item shows that he had become a high-profile figure. Their article, on 9 January 1968, was headlined 'Human Experiments Book Seized', and went on to explain that the issue probably centred on passages of the book 'which might be construed as allegations of manslaughter'. The *Daily Telegraph* took up the story on the same day: 'A City detective-sergeant is reading the book but before any decision is made about possible further action the author will be questioned. At present he is in the Far East'.

Despite his blackballing by the medical establishment, many in the profession were interested to hear more of Pappworth's views. Medical associations started inviting him to speak to students and those who taught them. In November 1967, for example, he was addressing the Manchester Medico-Ethical Association on the subject of 'Human Guinea Pigs;' nearly nine years later, in May 1976, he was back in Manchester, this time at the Polytechnic, in discussion with Dr L.A. Liversedge of the Manchester Royal Infirmary – once again on 'The Human Guinea Pig'.

Earlier, in 1970, despite the disapproval of consultants, junior doctors at the Hammersmith Hospital had invited Pappworth to be their guest speaker at one of their weekly talks. The evening passed harmoniously and was deemed a great success. *GP Magazine*, in its section 'The Enthusiasts' on 4 March 1977, ran a feature entitled 'Test Ban Treatment' on this legendary physician. Pappworth expressed his cynicism regarding the effectiveness of the ethical committees set up after *Human Guinea Pigs*' publication, also claiming that much of the correspondence from members of the public was from 'cranks'. But,' he added, 'that's what you'd expect.' He admitted that, ten years on from its original publication, *Human Guinea Pigs* was out of print, and likely to remain so. He observed to *GP*'s journalist that although colleagues criticised him for naming names, the book ruined no reputations. 'Many of the people I mentioned as culprits have achieved positions of distinction.'

Aged eighty, in 1990, Pappworth was asked to write an article for the *BMJ* on *Human Guinea Pigs*. He showed that he had remained true to the principles that had guided him throughout his career. Towards the end, he delivers one of his most unsettling denunciations: 'My opinion remains that those who dirty the linen and not those who wash it should be criticised. Some do not wash dirty linen in public or in private and the dirt is merely left to accumulate until it stinks.'

Professor Allan Gaw, who has championed Pappworth's work, points out that Pappworth is today 'largely forgotten', having failed to receive 'a single mention' in a 2008 textbook on clinical research ethics. Attacked in his lifetime, Pappworth was certainly not forgotten during it. He should be remembered now.

The student's candid friend: 'Passing Medical Examinations'

In 1972, with Pappworth a highly-respected and enticingly controversial figure, he was invited to speak to medical students in Dublin. From this lecture arose the last of his three books, *Passing Medical Examinations: A Guide to Undergraduates, Postgraduates and Examiners*, published by Butterworth in 1975 with a second edition appearing in 1985. It had originally been suggested by his brother A.D., who had noticed a similar book on passing law exams. The book is dedicated to 'my daughter Joanna' – possibly because I was almost the only member of the family with whom he was on speaking terms at this time. One can trace the fall-out of Pappworth family conflicts by noticing to whom each book and its subsequent editions are dedicated. He includes in this dedication the benediction from the prayer said in Jewish liturgy at the time of the New Moon. So he wishes me 'A long life; a life of peace, of good, of blessing, of sustenance, of bodily vigour; a life marked by the fear of Heaven and the dread of sin; a life free from shame and reproach; a life of prosperity and honour.' This beautiful prayer articulates a version of the life well lived, and one by which Pappworth himself doubtless wished to be remembered.

Pappworth had originally been invited not only to Dublin in 1972. Several Irish medical schools – in Belfast in Northern Ireland, and in the Irish Republic – had asked him to lecture, but it seemed impractical to get to all of them. So, as he explains in his Preface, he 'urged them to combine and arrange a joint meeting, preferably at University College, Dublin, because they had been the first to approach me'. All was agreed and arranged, and then a few days before the lecture Pappworth was asked to change its proposed title and instead to talk about passing final qualifying examinations. He was, after all, as famous for this expertise as for his controversial book of five years earlier. As it turned out, this event was to be – in Pappworth's own assessment of his life's work – one of the high points.

The year 1972 witnessed deep acrimony and serious violence in the struggle between Irish Protestants and Catholics in the North. In Dublin, he continues, 'The lecture was considered to have been a great success. Over 400 attended and, most important, probably for the first time in their long history, University College (a Catholic foundation) combined with Trinity College, Dublin (a Protestant foundation) in a joint meeting. Students also came from the Royal College of Surgeons (Dublin) and Galway Medical School and, most exciting of all, over forty came especially from Belfast. So I, a non-Christian, united Catholics and Protestants if only for one night. I shall always regard this as one of the highlights of my long career. This book is based on that, to me, memorable lecture… That meeting reinforced my belief that it is incumbent on everybody, whatever their religious belief or even if they are totally irreligious, to strive to establish the brotherhood of man, a principle which cannot be reconciled with racial or sectarian quarrels.'

Clearly very moved, Pappworth then appends three quotations. One is from Psalm 133, 'Behold, how good and how pleasant it is for brethren to dwell together in unity' (chanted during the Sabbath service); one from the prophet Malachi, 'Have not we all one Father? Did not God create us?'; finally, from St Paul's Epistle to the Romans, 'Be kindly and affectionate one to another with brotherly love.'

The first chapter of the book inspired by his Irish interlude of peace, *Passing Medical Examinations,* looks at 'The Purpose of Examinations'. Pappworth concedes that, certainly in the case of postgraduate exams, they serve to help make decisions about promotion. When students fail, he insists, the fault lies with their inadequate teachers, who have either neglected them or simply proved unable to teach. Like other senior physicians, he believes that the rather secretive Royal College of Physicians had 'made a mess' of its own examinations. Twelve years before this book's publication, the *BMJ* had printed a letter from Pappworth which asked pertinent questions about the College's plans for exam questions, examiners and the candidates' interpretation of statistics and technical procedures.

Later, *World Medicine*'s 'Talking Shop' feature in its September 1978 edition included the wittily titled 'Multiple Diplomatosis' by Maurice Pappworth, in which he recounts how he received an unsolicited prospectus for a diploma course in the Philosophy of Medicine, which he later reveals was organised by the Society of Apothecaries. Naturally, he was dubious about its value. In October and November 1980 the same journal published articles by Pappworth on, respectively, 'What Use Are Postgraduate Exams?' and 'How Not to Test Clinical Ability'. Medical education, like the ethics of research, continued to be of primary importance to him.

In *Passing Medical Examinations*, he points out that these tests are a money-spinner: without them, 'all the various medical colleges, royal and not so royal, would be very much poorer financially'. Not surprisingly, he disapproves of the recent growth in multiple choice tests. He was in all such matters a champion of the straightforward and conventional – although his suggestion that all potential examiners should pass an equivalent examination immediately prior to taking on the 'honour and responsibility' of becoming markers would have been deemed distinctly unorthodox. To the criticism that exams do not allow for original ideas, Pappworth's characteristic riposte is that 'Only a minute proportion of the population have ever had an original idea in their lives.'

Despite the faults of the current exam system, he acknowledges it as far better than a system of patronage, by which a consultant can 'make or break' the fortunes of a junior doctor. 'Dr Pimpernotta will get promotion to consultant rank merely because, and only if, his chief, Dr Scratchibaldi, with whom he has worked for several years, proclaims he should, and provided that Dr S, his chief, is influential and has very few enemies. Dr P will then get his promotion even if he has no higher qualifications, which are in themselves an indication that some outsiders (external examiners) as well as his chief have considered him capable and worthy of such promotion.'

Barely disguised, we have the story of that other Dr P, Dr Pappworth, who lacked the necessary chiefs and patrons during the early part of his career. Note that this key figure must have 'very few enemies'. This cannot have been said of his mentor Lord Cohen of Birkenhead, who later in the book he describes, with Professor Sir Arthur Hall of Sheffield, as two great and 'truly complete' physicians. We are back full circle with that awkward combination Pappworth encountered in his youthful job hunts: of anti-Semitism and anti-Cohenism.

Chapter Two, 'Preparations for Examination', provides interesting reading for a daughter of Maurice Pappworth. Although none of us went on to study medicine, he was full of advice and tips as we encountered school exams and university interviews. His maxim 'Do not exhibit a willingness to take everything from your teachers and parents except advice' rings still in my ears. Reading his words is like encountering a ghost. And when he warns his readers against 'the siren calls of permissiveness', I am taken back to the age in which I was a student, and my consciousness of his criticisms of society's collapsing moral fibre.

But his advice was often sound. He suggests that students should avoid studying at the weekend and, predictably, champions the usefulness of 'learning by rote', which had by the seventies become very unfashionable. He also suggests that students form 'quiz groups' to practise the art of verbal answers, but warns them to avoid including in their foursome 'smart alecs who insist in asking absurd or abstruse questions, often in an attempt to demonstrate their own supposed cleverness'. Pappworth hated the arrogance and pretentiousness of 'smart alecs'. He recommends the use of a tape recorder in preparing for oral examination: ask a friend or colleague to write down some suitable questions, which you should then tackle in your tape recording. Then it's time for feedback, when all your 'long periods of silence, wafflings and evasions, hesitations, lack of logical sequence of expression, frequent "ums" and "ers"…, poorness of elocution, and actual lack of knowledge of the subject, may all become apparent'. Pappworth could be brutal – but this was probably sound advice. It is a method of revision that has become increasingly popular through dictation straight into a mobile phone.

Chapter Four deals with 'Essay Questions', with a couple of *ad hominem* attacks on university professors whom he sees as responsible for the growing 'anti-essay' culture. Pappworth stresses the importance of 'the application and redaction of information which is scattered over many pages of several appropriate text-books'. His advice on writing examination answers is 'write a lot!' His conviction that many examiners marked questions by weight was one that several former students recall. Other recommendations which flew in the face of conventional wisdom include 'Planning answers is a grossly overrated and ill-advised exercise. Remember that you are not preparing a paper for publication in a learned journal.' He also suggests that candidates ignore 'the frequently given advice to always leave time to re-read your answers'. He warns against the use of abbreviations and of the pronouns 'I', 'we' or 'my'.

The chapter on the 'Oral Examination' sees Pappworth reminding students that 'your task in any oral is to keep on talking whenever allowed to do so.

Periods of silence must be avoided at all costs… Start talking right away and hope further inspiration will come as you proceed.' The Pappworth formula does not seem well fitted for the thoughtful candidate who likes to work out a measured judgement in advance. But there is good sense in the advice to avoid mumbling and to 'talk a little louder than you ordinarily do'. In formal situations Pappworth certainly followed his own advice, his lectures being delivered at several decibels above the norm, with slow emphasis and with a rolling of his 'r's. 'The three C's – Clarity, Conciseness and Confidence – must always be your aim.' This use of alliteration in helping candidates to remember was a strong feature of his own spoken rhetorical style.

Whatever one might think of Pappworth's suggested routes to success, the student reader of *Passing Medical Examinations* would have understood that its author was on their side, just as his MRCP students did. He was trying to prepare them for and protect them from 'examiners who seem to gain a sadistic pleasure in destroying a candidate's morale'. But he is keen that any sense of confrontation should not cause the candidate to make lapses in etiquette: 'You should insert the occasional judiciously placed "sir" (or "madam") without appearing to be unduly grovelling,' and, at the end, a 'thank you' to the examiner which at least tries to sound sincere leaves a positive final impression.

It is this attention to apparently trivial but useful detail which makes the book very much a product of the Pappworth mind. In the chapter on 'Clinical Examinations', he advises candidates to bring their own instruments, giving detailed advice on these. He recommends that female candidates avoid carrying their instruments in a 'psychedelically embellished' bag. Another evocative example of those exciting times! His further advice that 'cosmetics and perfumes must be used sparingly, and nail varnish is usually frowned upon' once again takes me back to his standards when his daughters were teenagers and in their early twenties. I can recall him walking me to the front gate one evening when I was setting off on a date. He stopped, inhaled, and remarked, 'Overdone it on the perfume a bit, haven't you?' He expressed huge pride in the fact that Dinah got married 'without a trace of make-up on her face'.

When turning to male candidates, Pappworth acknowledges – again summoning up the early seventies – that 'It is now fashionable to have long hair but, however much it may offend your ego, however much you may resent interference with your personal freedom of choice, you must pocket your pride and get your hair cut a few days before the [oral] examination.' Thus the man who was such a champion of the patient's 'personal freedom of choice' could compartmentalise his views, and understand when these freedoms mattered – and when they didn't.

More practical advice is on hand in the chapter on 'The Long Case – History-Taking'. Pappworth describes as 'essential', given the limited time at his disposal, the need for the candidate to try to get on good terms with the patient right from the start. 'Your approach must be continually friendly, sympathetic, warm, kindly, generous, good-mannered and humble, and never arrogant'. That is a long list of adjectives for the nervous candidate to keep in mind. Pappworth underlines the importance of learning from the patient, as quickly as possible, his main symptoms. He then goes into great detail about how the questioning should proceed. He specifies how long should be spent on history-taking, once you know how much time you have got for the long case. 'Getting a history and doing a physical examination should always be regarded as a continuous process and never as two completely distinct... activities.' Explaining his reasoning, he points out that the physical examination may reveal symptoms which make you want to ask further questions of the patient.

Once again, Pappworth dismisses what many of his colleagues recommend: 'The commonly given advice that you should allow patients to tell their story in their own way and in their own time with little or no interruption is impracticable and bad advice for any clinical examination. With some patients, in the time allowed you would not complete even the history, let alone the physical examination as well. Careful guiding and polite interruptions are usually essential.'

It is said that if you keep the patient talking for long enough, he will reveal his diagnosis. This may well be true, but Pappworth keeps attention on the fact that such a method will not work in the time-strapped context of the long case, and gives advice on which 'leading questions' to ask. In the physical examination, he emphasises that all systems must be examined. Other useful tips include examining the patient 'from above downwards, and do not automatically start with the part of the anatomy about which the patient is complaining.'

More basic but equally important advice is offered on the subject of undressing. Obviously the patient will need to remove clothes but, as in his MRCP lectures, Pappworth tries to instil empathy, to make students realise that in matters of personal dignity the patient must always be treated with tact and care. Finally, Pappworth provides three key questions which should be asked of the patient at the end of the long case, and recommends leaving at least three minutes' pause to consider how best to present the history and physical diagnosis, and what questions you are likely to be asked.

Pappworth informs his readers that, for the short cases, about five minutes each is allowed. 'Speed then becomes the essence of the best.' Once again, Pappworth uses his 'wide-angle lenses' phrase, the doctor's eyes being described here as 'God-given'. He lists thirteen rules which candidates should follow when undertaking the short cases: this part of the examination could create great pressure. Quoting from the Viennese writer Stefan Zweig's memoir The *World of Yesterday*, he reminds them that 'The eternal secret of all great art, yes, of every mortal achievement, is concentration.' This concentration must not lapse when it comes to 'Relations with Examiners'. As with the patient, it is 'obligatory' to remain on good terms with examiners. Pappworth warns against any display of anxiety or 'fright', and advises, 'Always conceal your mistakes and your difficulties and hope that you will not be found out.' Like his advice to his MRCP students to pretend they know about some obscure nineteenth-century doctor, this is a typical Pappworth line.

Senior tutor – and veteran trouble-maker

Pappworth continued to take an interest in medical education. A brick wall had greeted his 1963 letter to the *BMJ*, challenging the College of General Practitioners to consider suitable cases and questions for their proposed examination, asking who the examiners were to be, and wondering how much importance would be attached to a knowledge of technical diagnostic tools such as ECGs and radiology. Pappworth remained frustrated but unsurprised by the fact that, despite his many admirers, the medical élite maintained its policy of ignoring him. Fourteen years later, in his interview with *GP* Magazine, he admitted that he would love to compensate what he still considered to be the poor quality of medical teaching by himself teaching undergraduates 'before they get contaminated', in addition to postgraduates. His requests to do so were apparently turned down because he was not 'the right type'. The oft-mentioned 'establishment,' claims the reporter, 'obviously does not forgive.'

During October and November 1980, *World Medicine* published a series of three articles by Pappworth on postgraduate training. Here Pappworth traces the founding of the Royal College of Physicians in the sixteenth century and the introduction of the Membership examination in 1859. Unusually for him, he names no names, but claims that several doctors, having repeatedly failed the exam, were later awarded it 'by some back door', subsequently being elected to a Fellowship and even becoming examiners for the MRCP 'when they themselves had failed to pass'. He highlights the exclusiveness of the College by his revelation that the examination included an optional paper with passages of Latin, Greek, French and German for translation. These were not fully discontinued until the mid-1950s. Not surprisingly, this scholarly exercise being optional, Pappworth advised candidates to spend their time instead on improving their compulsory essays. He continued to express his contempt for multiple choice questions, describing them as a 'parasitic fungus eroding medical education'. There are those in many branches of education today who would appreciate his metaphor.

Pappworth continued to write almost until the end of his life. *Passing Medical Examinations* went into a second edition, though he was disappointed that the fifth edition of his *Primer of Medicine* was not, in the words of Charles Fry, publishing director of Butterworths, 'selling as fast as the previous edition did at this stage in its life'. Writing to the author on 15 February 1989, Fry requests some 'sample pages' of work in progress for the new edition of the *Primer* that Pappworth was planning. In a letter written two and a half years previously, Fry had predicted that although two thousand five hundred copies of the latest *Primer* had been sold, with almost that number still remaining in stock it would be a further two years before a reprint could be issued. This, in the view of the canny publisher, would be preferable to an entire 'revamp'. The 'couple of years' suggested had more than passed, and it was clear that Butterworths were putting on the back burner ideas of a sixth edition.

In his 1989 letter, Fry reassures Pappworth that *Passing Medical Examinations* 'is also doing quite nicely, although again there is no rush to contemplate a new edition'. Two thousand six hundred copies had apparently been sold; 1,400 were yet to be bought, which meant that a new edition couldn't be contemplated for another three years. But time was marching on for the doctor with heart disease. Fry alludes to this condition when, at the end of his letter, he expresses sympathy for Pappworth's 'further set-backs to your health', adding emolliently that the publishers 'have every confidence in you retaining your reputation as one of our most enduring authors'.

Another of Pappworth's projects was a book on coronary disease aimed at the lay reader, which his New York friend Dr Dennis Bloomfield would co-author. But a letter sent to him by Fry at the end of August 1987 dealt this one a blow: it was 'something we could not do justice to'. Clearly, if the book was going to see the light of day, Pappworth would have to find a different publisher, and one which did not specialise in professional textbooks. Fry suggested a couple of alternatives, including Oxford University Press. But the public was to remain deprived of Pappworth's expertise (both as physician and patient) on coronary disease. One suspects that these days the outcome would be very different, as public interest in particular diseases has led to some very successful books for a lay audience.

Setbacks continued. Aware that his deteriorating health created a certain urgency to his plans, Pappworth was keen to pursue work on his other proposed book – on medical aphorisms, a favourite topic. In 1987 Butterworths had expressed interest in such a book, and requested some samples. Judging by the papers Pappworth left in his study (by now, his workplace was what had once been Jean's specially-built studio in the garden), he does not seem to have succeeded in making much progress. He was elderly; he was tired; myocardial infarction seemed to be taking him with increased frequency to the Royal Free. In a letter dated 13 February 1990, Charles Fry continued to go out of his way to maintain good relations with this distinguished, difficult and disappointed author, thoughtfully but erroneously congratulating him on 'achieving your three score years and ten' when Pappworth had just turned eighty. 'I am sorry,' he wrote, 'to hear you have not been well but from the tone of your letter you sound cheerful, and if your desire to get on with new editions of your books is anything to go by your appetite for life is undiminished.' But he then goes on to admit that, with sales of the *Primer* having diminished to about one hundred and fifty a year, and with a thousand copies still in stock, there was little chance of a reprint, let alone a new edition.

During Pappworth's last two decades, he continued to be a figure of interest to the press – though he doubtless felt a little uneasy to find himself featuring twice in the *News of the World*. In March 1972, under the blaring headline 'Storm Over New Sex Tests', the tabloid ran an article on a recently-conducted experiment aimed at 'solving a man's sexual problems'. The reporter, David Roxan, interviewed both the experimenter, Dr Robert Heath, and also of course the 'leading campaigner against the use of human guinea-pigs,' Dr Maurice Pappworth. Two and a half years later, the *News of the World*'s Pappworth story, headed 'Doctor Raps the £10,000 Consultants', focused on top doctors who were earning more than £10,000 a year for National Health Service work that amounted to only four or five hours a week, then proceeding to use NHS doctors and equipment for 'private operations in private clinics'. The source was that 'leading campaigner against human guinea-pig experiments in hospital,' Dr Maurice Pappworth – who, the report adds, 'treats only private patients'. Pappworth was objecting to the use of private beds on hard-pressed NHS wards. But doctors were warning they would go on strike if Social Services Secretary Barbara Castle modified her plans to end pay-beds in public hospitals.

Pappworth's strong feelings on this matter were confirmed to me by Dr Guy Staight, whose decision to go immediately into private practice received approbation from his former teacher. In the press, the story rumbled on, the start of 1975 bringing an article for the *Times* by M.H. Pappworth on 'Get-rich Doctors Who Exploit the Health Service'. Pappworth expanded on the abuses practised by hospital consultants, who were not working the number of hours they were contracted to by the NHS but instead used NHS facilities – not just hospital beds, but also intensive care, X-rays and therapies, all provided by NHS staff – to treat their private patients. Junior doctors frequently undertook the surgery and anaesthetics that consultants were unable to conduct, being away at medical conferences or on their six weeks' annual leave.

Pappworth stressed that such consultants were in a minority, but called for strong action against those who did milk the system. He was also indignant at the 'merit award' distributed secretly each year to consultants, with no public control in place. The £1,250 to £7,500 per annum a doctor might receive rarely went to those working in 'the least salubrious' parts of the country' or in 'less glamorous specialities' such as mental disease and geriatrics. Writing for *World Medicine* in October 1980 in an article entitled 'Merit Awards and Human Guinea Pigs', Pappworth assured Professor David Kerr, who had challenged him to cut his own income: 'I am proud to proclaim that I have never been involved in the clandestine and sordid manoeuvres to grab public money.' If anything, Pappworth was becoming still more political as he approached old age. He continued to enjoy a certain prominence in sections of the press. Whenever a controversial medical topic cropped up in the news, Maurice Pappworth was their man.

He carried on writing articles for medical journals. *World Medicine* appears to have been a favourite. For them he contributed a humorous article on one of his pet subjects, 'Medical Vocabulary' (1977). The following year the same journal printed two detailed, more conventionally clinical pieces – on 'Diagnosing Angina Pectoris' (featuring rather a good photo of the author) and 'Ptosis' (the photograph being of the poet Dame Edith Sitwell, who suffered from this drooping upper eyelid condition – although Pappworth later complained that the picture was 'inappropriate' and did not in fact illustrate ptosis.) He forgave them sufficiently to contribute further articles including, in March 1982, a scholarly but very readable one on Down's Syndrome: 'Was Down a Racist?'

World Medicine recognised that in Pappworth they could be sure of a writer who provided lively, informative articles on subjects that would catch their readers' attention. Arguably, this was more his type of forum than the sedate *BMJ* or *Lancet*. So the Sitwell-embellished piece was followed in October 1978 by Pappworth's opinions on 'The Penis in Chinese Therapy'. This gave the author a chance to air his contempt for alternative medicine, in this case of the Chinese variety. He lists the ingredients of one particularly popular drug produced in China by a large pharmaceutical company, evidently aimed at those worried about their sexual performance: these included antler extract and the penises of deer, donkey and dog.

'He never gave a sense of caring': against Freud and the psychoanalysts

Having reached this part of the anatomy, now might be the time to consider the role played by Sigmund Freud in the life of Maurice Pappworth. It was an indirect role, but significant, as Maurice's wife Jean spent many years in psychoanalysis. By the time she met her future husband, she had been analysed by the great man's daughter, Anna Freud (after whom, as my mother informed me, she named me). She continued to visit a number of psychoanalysts and psychotherapists as she found herself increasingly unhappy in her marriage. But for Maurice, Freudian psychoanalysis was like traditional Chinese medicine: a scam which exploited the vulnerable.

Between 1975 and 1976, *MIMS Magazine* (which specialises in providing health professionals with information about prescription medicines) published three articles by Pappworth on the subject of psychoanalysis. These forcefully articulate his objections to this type of psychiatric treatment. In the first, he compares psychoanalysis to 'that other mumbojumbo' Scientology, likewise described as a brainwashing cult. Pappworth constantly had an eye on such organisations. He admitted to me late in his life that he had been visited by a so-called academic researcher who claimed, like him, to be investigating the cult of the Moonies. It is a mark of Pappworth's naivety that he handed this young man all the work for his own proposed exposé of the Moonies. Predictably, his visitor turned out to be one of them. Pappworth never tilted at windmills: all the targets of his criticism genuinely needed to be challenged. It is interesting, nonetheless, that there was always something that seemed to be waiting there for him to attack.

Pappworth explains that psychoanalysis is 'merely an esoteric form of psychotherapy – the treatment of mental and emotional disturbances by talking'. Early on he dismisses the Oedipus complex as 'a product of bourgeois old Vienna': Oedipus himself, but also Freud, lacked the presence of their natural mother during their upbringing. For Freud, it had not been abandonment on a mountainside but the substitution of a nanny. You are unlikely to want to marry your mother if you have been close since infancy.

It is easy now to ridicule Freudian theory, long after its British heyday in the immediate post-war decades. But Pappworth, always one to point out that the emperor was wearing no clothes, was bold in deriding Freud's 'insistence on the domination of every infant's emotion development by sexual instincts and frustrations'. This leads to 'a narrow determinism in which all achievements are reduced to the lowest sexual factors', and 'allows no room for human aspirations, goodness, spirituality, romance or altruism'. Freudian doctrine reduces 'the whole of human endeavour to basic aggressions and sexual drives of a most primitive kind. Psychoanalysis is a militant irrational religious cult.'

A particular flaw in psychoanalysis was its anti-religious stance. 'I object to psychoanalysis,' proclaims Pappworth, unlike Freud a practising Jew, 'both on religious grounds because it adversely affects free will, and moral grounds because it diminishes the sense of responsibility and may break down defence mechanisms which normally inhibit foolish and wrong actions.' In the second article he accuses psychoanalysts of 'dulling' the conscience, and the 'shameless encouragement of an almost lascivious preoccupation with self.' As he reminded readers of a piece he wrote at this time for his synagogue magazine, 'Judaism teaches self-restraint, and one of its fundamental beliefs is in… each individual being responsible for his own actions. Freud taught that man is… shackled by biological urges… Judaism rests on faith – faith in an omnipotent and omniscient God. Psychoanalysts are completely lacking in faith, except in the Freudian version of the self.' It is ironic that, as he pointed out to his fellow congregants, over seventy-five per cent of psychoanalysts during the 1960s and 1970s were of Jewish extraction. He claimed to know many of them, and found those with whom he discussed religious matters to be 'proud atheists, strongly hostile to all organised religions'.

Pappworth also objects to the physical and mental distance placed between therapist and patient, as this runs counter to his own beliefs about the doctor-patient relationship. 'Freud seemed to me to be a bad doctor because he revealed no close sympathy with his patients. He never gave a sense of caring.' One of his many objections to psychoanalysis was that its primary aim seemed to have little to do with actually providing a cure. Many of the cases seen by psychoanalysts were simply unhappy. Pappworth claimed that psychoanalysts 'have made unhappiness a disease entity and ignore the fact that very few people go through life without ever being unhappy.'

Practitioners claim that they give the patient 'a new deep inner understanding of himself,' but all too often, according to Pappworth, the end product is someone filled with self-pity, and blaming others – notably his parents – for his woes. He declares that 'Psychoanalysis diverts patients from facing their problems and learning from their experiences – the best ways of resolving inner conflict.'

Pappworth was, in many ways, a man riven by this condition. I remember him, towards the end of his life, sitting in his black leather Eames armchair in the sitting room of Vale Lodge, listening to Brahms' fourth symphony. This, so my father told me, was music on the theme of 'tragic conflict'. Maybe this is how he solved his inner turmoil, especially after he had been left alone. He always enjoyed music, despite his off-key singing voice. At the very end, his preference shifted to chamber music.

Then, of course, there was the financial side. In January 1975 he had written an article for the *Times* on the irregularities of some consultants' earnings. Now, in October, we have him pointing out that the Psychoanalytical Association recommends to its members that they charge £10 to £15 for each of five hourly sessions per week – in other words £2,000 to £3,700 per annum (£15,000 to £28,000 at 2016 values). 'A psychoanalyst thus needs only six patients to earn a good living and then to make him wealthy.' With a kind of dour grimace, he continues, 'I am assured that the hour is nearly always accurately timed. Indeed there are recorded reports of Freud himself interrupting patients in mid-sentence and abruptly stopping the session when the hour was up.' He reminds readers that lay psychoanalysts (who practise the therapy alongside qualified psychiatrists) have received no medical training 'outside the straitjacket of psychoanalysis'. This can lead to tragedy, as in the case of composer George Gershwin who, suffering from persistent headaches, consulted an analyst. It was only after a year of 'probing into his "infantile sexuality"' that he sought advice from a neurologist. By then his meningioma (a type of brain tumour) had grown significantly, and he did not survive its attempted removal.

Pappworth condemns psychoanalysis as 'an élitist therapy' in which the chief criterion in the selection of patients is their ability to pay. Now there are opportunities to receive psychoanalytical treatment through the National Health Service, and it is more readily available countrywide. Pappworth's researches in the mid-1970s revealed that only fourteen of the 175 medically qualified practitioners recognised by the Institute of Psychoanalysis lived and worked outside the Greater London area. And of the ninety-one lay psychoanalysts, only two practised outside London. Strikingly, eighty-two psychoanalysts lived at the time in Hampstead (home of Sigmund and Anna) and ten in St John's Wood. The persistence with which he gathered these figures indicates Pappworth's increasing impatience with the exclusivity of this type of treatment, while the expense involved fed into its apparent indifference to effecting a cure. A senior psychoanalyst privately informed him that he saw no problem with the concept of never-ending 'treatment,' maintaining that if a patient feels he needs a 'crutch', he should be given one permanently. But as Pappworth points out, it is the surgeon's duty to persuade their patients to 'discard their crutches as soon as possible; otherwise they will never recover'.

A final reason for Pappworth's distrust lay in his interest in education. He expressed contempt for 'permissiveness', and this attitude he blames partly on Freud's views: these, he insisted, had created 'disastrous' effects at all levels of education. He attributes to Freud 'the idea that children should be brought up in a moral vacuum and should acquire their own values and judgements as they mature.' This unfortunately guarantees that 'they will grow up without genuine ethical values'.

His interpretation of psychoanalysis is that it demands that 'nobody, least of all parents and teachers, has the right to even ask for obedience, let alone demand it'. This was naturally discordant with the Pappworth view that 'to be effective, education must be backed to some degree by authority'. He continues: 'In my view, children should be brought up to know and appreciate that obedience to parents and teachers leads to harmony and happiness.' These certainly sound like words of a man who at the time had three daughters in their late teens and early twenties, for whom the notion of obedience to a rather exacting father was now brazenly flouted. When he caught me revising for my history O level over a Jewish festival, my father confiscated my books and files, asserting that my headmistress would concur. Children should always obey their parents.

For Pappworth, psychoanalysis was in essence a fashionable and expensive form of confession. To his critics, this preoccupation would represent yet another bee in the Pappworth bonnet. But it is undeniable that Jean's long-term reliance on psychoanalysis drove a wedge between himself and her. Predictably, she was told by her analyst to be more assertive. This was at odds with Pappworth's outlook, which contained a curious blend of ambition for his daughters and a traditional Jewish view of the self-sacrificing wife. His mother, the ultimate '*ayshet chayil*', had provided the perfect model.

Chapter Eight

Gratitude and solitude: a prophet honoured and a man alone

'This little man shuffled up to get his Fellowship, and applause broke out. It was very moving. A wrong was being righted.'

(Dr David London, Registrar of the Royal College of Physicians, on the award of the College's Fellowship to Maurice Pappworth in 1993)

End of a Marriage

Keen to show his family the Old City of Jerusalem, Pappworth took his daughters in spring 1971 on a holiday to Israel. Our mother decided not to join us, opting instead for a cruise of the eastern Mediterranean. As our father revealed to her shocked Israeli friends (whose company she would definitely have preferred to a cruise – the only one she ever took), it included a stop-off in Libya. Jean was sadly cutting off her nose to spite her face. Not long afterwards, Maurice returned from a trip to the Far East with his brother A.D. (Jean refused that one as well) to find that she had moved out of the marital bedroom and into a lovely, sun-filled little room on the third floor of Vale Lodge in Hampstead – formerly the au pair's bedroom.

My childhood nights had been punctuated by the sound of my parents' rows (my bedroom adjoined theirs). Many, it appears, were about such trivial topics as whether or not to have the curtains, as well as the windows, open. So it came as something of a relief to me when my mother moved upstairs. I once overheard what was definitely an act of violence, the sudden thud being a giveaway, but there was no physical evidence the following morning. I had no sense that our father made a habit of physical aggression against his wife – or, indeed, any of his children.

Family life continued in this strained atmosphere, with the lack of verbal communication between our parents as unnerving to the three girls as the regular open rows. Then we started to drift away. After leaving school in 1972, I travelled across the United States, where I encountered the American contingent of the Papperovitch clan. In October of the following year I started at my aunt Naomi's Oxford *alma mater*, St Hugh's. Both parents accompanied me and spent a night at the Randolph Hotel, which indicates some attempt to present a normal façade to their daughter, and also perhaps a wish to share their pride in my achievement.

It was during my time at Oxford that, from a distance, I could sense the marriage enter its final stage of disintegration. Although there was no talk of divorce, I did receive a letter from my father asking me to write to my mother's solicitor to put his side of the case. Jean, on the other hand, never involved her children in her marital disharmony in such a demanding fashion. I do remember her once sitting at the end of my bed and bursting into tears, sobbing with grief. I am ashamed to say I proved myself a true Pappworth, finding it impossible to cover her with the physical affection she so craved.

Maurice never displayed his emotions in this way, but he talked to me a great deal. He anointed the precious eldest daughter with the bitter oil of his sorrows – every last drop of it, so it seemed. He had by now few close friends with whom he could talk on such matters, whereas our mother, who had a great capacity for friendship, was never short of sympathetic ears. It was indeed an unfortunate story. His best friend and best man, Sidney Nathan, died young. Not long after this, another close friend, Philip Druiff, died suddenly. Maurice also felt wary of inviting friends to our house. All went well with when it came to the two doctor friends with whose sons we enjoyed playing: our mother liked both families. But, whether reasonably or not, Maurice felt that his wife could not be relied upon to provide the necessary welcome to his guests. So he tended to socialise away from home, with a favourite meeting place the doctors' 'club'. The Royal Society of Medicine.

It is striking how many of Maurice's close friends suffered from problems of their own: there was the alcoholic, the husband of a mentally ill wife, the father of sons addicted to drugs and alcohol, the father whose son was murdered. Something in him appears to have attracted the vulnerable. That must be one of the many reasons why he was such a good bedside physician.

Jean was financially independent, which enabled her to plan her escape carefully in advance. She had already purchased a little Victorian terraced house in Gospel Oak, on its way to becoming a fashionable oasis of northwest London. In April 1975, Jean moved out of Vale Lodge and into her new home. I was in my second year at university; Dinah was on a leadership training programme in Israel; Sara would in a few months' time be leaving South Hampstead to take her A levels at another school. She decided to stay with what was familiar, but eventually chose to live with her mother. When Sara left Vale Lodge, her cat Sacha accompanied her. Unfortunately, Sacha's feline attachment to place meant that, when it came to dinner-time, his former abode was where he needed to be. It became a fairly regular evening occurrence during the first months after her departure for Maurice to telephone his estranged wife and announce 'The cat's here'. In his own version of 'The Incredible Journey,' Sacha had crossed Hampstead Heath to present himself at the back door for feeding.

Maurice and Jean never divorced. Neither of them found another partner. The mutual decision to remain separated rather than to break the legal tie will have arisen partly from their joint wish to have as little to do with each other as possible, and also from financial considerations. My father never came to terms with the situation. 'You could have knocked me down with a feather,' he told my parents-in-law about ten years later when discussing Jean's announcement that she was leaving him. Of course, he had seen the writing on the wall, but it seems to have been a matter of pride for him to keep people in the dark about the true state of affairs. During the late 1970s, we were visited by a former au pair girl and also the rabbi who had officiated at his wedding. Both were told that Jean was 'away'. I felt embarrassed – and also ashamed at silently colluding in this story.

Maurice became quite competent at cooking for himself, although he would have been completely at sea without the devoted oversight of his sister Esther, who always came in on wash day. She also helped Maurice with his shopping, and was even known to take his dog to the vet. This enormous but gentle-natured Old English mastiff was already called Simon when he joined the family. It was the name our parents planned to give the son who never showed up. Once Jean, Sara and Sacha had left, this was Maurice's one companion. Our mother (who was actually very attached to him) dismissed Simon as 'a status dog'. Dad's primary reason for choosing this breed was that he hoped it would be an effective guard dog, and both parents were looking for a dog that didn't require much walking. This was strange reasoning, as they were both keen walkers and our house bordered Hampstead Heath. As a result we all over-walked Simon and his predecessor, Caius, who died early of hip dysplasia. These two mastiffs could not have been more different from the motley Jacky of Maurice's Birkenhead childhood.

A patriarch and his daughters

The March 1977 profile of Dr Maurice Pappworth in *GP* magazine was spread over two pages, including photographs that captured the subject's personality. Its tone borders on the reverential, and offers an interesting impression of what a visitor to Vale Lodge might conclude. The profile opens thus: 'Maurice Pappworth is a small, neat man in his late 60s with fast yet purposeful movements. He exudes an air of contentment and unflamboyant conviction which one cannot help admiring. Matter-of-fact rather than didactic, he never smiles superfluously, yet the deep lines round his eyes show that, despite his crusading image, Dr Pappworth is not an earnest man.' Of course, this reporter had no idea that the 'small building which could easily be mistaken for a summer house or greenhouse', from which Pappworth now conducted his private practice, was once upon a time the studio of his estranged wife. 'The Pappworth home,' we are told, 'is large and airy but the affluence is understated.'

Pappworth's 'oddly ambivalent position in medical circles' is summed up by his alienation from 'the establishment' as opposed to the respect awarded him for his diagnostic brilliance. Without conceit, apparently, he claimed 'I can give a lecture on bone X-rays and then talk about skin disease and then deal with neurology.' He was undoubtedly proud to be able to set himself apart from the 'super-specialists' who, then as now, dominated clinical medicine.

Hidden from others' eyes were more personal concerns. By the mid-1970s, his daughters' boyfriends had become a hot topic for Dr Pappworth. No-one was going to be good enough for any of us. Sometimes we simply resorted to secrecy. In the early 1980s, I heard my father give a lecture on diagnosis, in which he stressed the importance of recognising a patient's emotional state. He cited the case of a university student who developed acute stomach pains. It transpired that these were caused by anxiety about her forthcoming examinations. 'That young woman,' he concluded dramatically, 'was none other than my own daughter.' Sitting in the audience, her eldest sister was aware that Sara's physical symptoms were caused as much – if not more – by problems with her current boyfriend than exam worries. But Sara had taken care that our father should know nothing about this relationship.

Dinah possibly fared best on the approval ratings, as the only daughter to marry someone whose roots were entirely Jewish. She and Saul (always known by the family as 'Buck') had met in Israel during her gap year. He hailed from Texas, but followed Dinah to Cambridge where he enrolled at what was then the Cambridgeshire College of Arts and Technology (now part of Anglia Ruskin University) in order to be close to his beloved. Maurice was visibly happy at Dinah and Buck's wedding in a garden in Ein Kerem, the village just outside Jerusalem where they lived at the time, in October 1980. Then he proudly acted as 'Sandak' (the Jewish version of a godfather, who holds the male baby during the circumcision ceremony) to his first grandchild. Amos was born in Jerusalem in December 1984.

During my last year at Oxford I started going out with a law student. Like my father, Alex was a Cheshire lad, brought up in Bebington and an alumnus of the Wirral Grammar School. However, they had little in common. Alex's visits to Vale Lodge were invariably tense occasions. Sharing the Sabbath dinner with my father and me, the boyfriend revealed his awareness that two forms of grace after meals – always recited in Hebrew, of course – existed: the traditional grace and a shorter form. While I was preparing to do the honours, my father noticed Alex raising his hands, fingers together, and moving them towards each other. He understood immediately that our guest was silently requesting me to opt for the shorter form, and was not amused.

I still have a typed letter my father wrote to me, probably in 1977. The context was my refusal to join him on a trip to the Jewish centres of medieval Spain. Tactlessly, I pointed out that I had recently been there with Alex – and in any case, I remember writing, there was no point in my going as long as he openly opposed our relationship. My father's response opens formally: 'Your letter was received and its contents noted.' Then follows the anger and unhappiness of a man whose daughter had, like his wife, abandoned him in the quest for her own path in life. 'I am shocked and profoundly chagrined and upset that you continue your association with Alex.' He concludes with the words 'Love to you, my clever but very silly daughter.' It is clear from the signature that he had started to write 'MHP', but spotted his error and changed the M to the D of 'Dad.'

Alex moved to California, to study film at UCLA, and a transatlantic relationship looked impossible to maintain. Three months later, I started going out with Anthony, whom I had known since the summer term of our first year at Oxford. His father, the economist Arthur Seldon, was, like Maurice, from an immigrant Jewish family. They had come from Ukraine and settled in the East End. There was tragedy also in that family: both parents died during the Spanish Flu epidemic after the First World War, leaving five orphaned children.

Arthur, the baby, was adopted by a childless and impoverished Jewish couple. Like Maurice, he was determined to better himself through education and hard work. He married Marjorie Willett, Christian by birth but secular by inclination, and gradually distanced himself from his Jewish roots. He had sung in the synagogue choir as a boy but until, at the end of his life, he became interested once again in the religion and joined our progressive synagogue in Brighton, his attitude to his Jewish identity could not have been more different from my father's. Anthony, the youngest of the couple's three sons, was confirmed in Tonbridge School Chapel.

Maurice first encountered Arthur and Marjorie when they turned up at Heathrow Airport in October 1980 to give Anthony and me a lift home on our return from Dinah's wedding. This was, for me, unusual treatment: I cannot remember my parents ever meeting me off an aeroplane. (When I went out on a Saturday night as a teenager, my parents never picked me up.) Anthony and I emerged through customs, accompanying my father. Immediately, Arthur and Marjorie offered Maurice a lift to his home. To drive from Heathrow to Sevenoaks via Hampstead was something of a diversion, but it was typical of the Seldons' kindness to think of doing so.

Maurice was placed in a real quandary. He didn't approve of this non-Jewish boyfriend of mine. According to Orthodox Judaism the line is matrilineal so, despite his Jewish father, Anthony was a 'goy', a non-Jew. For Maurice, naturally, the last thing he should do was to show the slightest sign of a positive attitude. He should take the Underground – but there was Arthur's Jaguar, gleaming in the car park. The temptation was too great. Maurice accepted the lift in the smart car of his daughter's non-Jewish boyfriend's parents. Throughout the journey, he uttered not a word. Later, this being his habit, his iciness thawed. He ended up growing close to Arthur and Marjorie. They would invite him to their garden parties in Sevenoaks, and loved nothing more than to talk medicine with him.

My father insisted that, if Anthony and I were to marry, the bridegroom needed to convert to Judaism before the wedding. So my family history turned an interesting circle. I became a member of the West London Synagogue, the Reform synagogue where my mother's grandparents had been members and leaders. Anthony underwent a course of instruction there. Partners were required to attend, and I learned a great deal. We were married in July 1982 by Hugo Gryn, the charismatic rabbi who had survived Theresienstadt and Auschwitz, losing both his father and brother. He had been an enormous source of comfort to my maternal grandparents as they approached their deaths. Anthony and I loved him, as did so many. Even my father approved – though he did once write to Hugo pointing out that he had, on BBC Radio 4's 'Thought for the Day', mistakenly attributed to the prophet Amos the words of Micah. The pedagogue in Dr Maurice Pappworth could never resist correcting errors. My mother was very anxious before the wedding, writing to Maurice imploring that they behave in a 'civilised' manner towards each other on this special day. She received no reply. He could be totally unforgiving.

Maurice certainly showed himself to be unforgiving in his treatment of Sara, his youngest daughter. Present at Anthony's and my wedding was the man Sara would marry three years later. Nick was a lapsed-Catholic atheist. Maurice objected less to his Catholic upbringing (which showed, after all, that his childhood had been rooted in a traditional religion) than to Nick's conscious decision to become an atheist. Ironically, as a geneticist heavily involved in research, Nick worked at none other than Pappworth's hated Hammersmith Hospital.

Maurice didn't attend Sara's wedding and cut himself off completely from her. He loved my three children, and took great pleasure in our visits from south of the Thames. But he never met Sara's two sons (her daughter Katie was born after his death), who lived not far from him, until six months before he died. When he told his sister Naomi that he intended to have nothing more to do with Sara and her family, she told him not to be such 'a bloody fool'. Naomi took his response literally: 'Never darken my door again'. Maurice's world, through his own destructive and self-destructive obstinacy, was fast becoming smaller. His courage in publishing *Human Guinea Pigs* revealed Maurice Pappworth as a man of enormous principle. The trouble with people of principle is that, when this trait spills over into their personal lives, the effects can be terribly damaging.

Maurice's solitary life, marked by the routines of the elderly, carried on, punctuated by the misbehaviour of his heart and also by spurts of energy. He continued to write letters and articles, and was quite frequently asked to review medical books. Thanks to his friend Stuart MacPherson's contacts in Malaysia and other countries in the Far East, Maurice travelled to this part of the world so long as his health permitted, delivering lectures in Kuala Lumpur and Hong Kong. He was treated like royalty, and assured me that I would experience the same if I accompanied him to Kuala Lumpur. I still regret having rejected his offer. It was ungracious, and must have hurt my father deeply.

In his late seventies, he travelled to Mauritius to see patients and deliver a lecture. He also lectured in New York, Chicago, New Orleans and Arizona, and in Israel in Jerusalem and Beersheba. Closer to home, he lectured at teaching hospitals in Edinburgh and Glasgow. While he and Jean were still together, they had travelled to Iran shortly before the fall of the Shah: he had been made a visiting professor at both Shiraz and Teheran universities. He was always curious and open to different cultures – partly because he felt so confidently rooted in his own.

His nineteen post-Jean years at Vale Lodge were not entirely spent alone. Apart from sporadic stays by his daughters, there was the A.D. experiment. After the death of his sister Rivkah, who had looked after her brother in Birkenhead, A.D. was rather a lost soul. The family's eldest brother had always hankered after a life in London, an ambition thwarted by Rivkah's antipathy to the south. It was agreed that A.D. should live with Maurice at Vale Lodge. For Esther, this was delightful: she could now look after two of her brothers. But the experiment was not a success. A.D. had never done anything practical for himself, and was totally undomesticated. Now he found himself living in a house where he was expected to contribute to the shopping, cooking and washing up. Maurice interpreted his unhelpfulness as laziness – though the poor man was probably floundering on alien seas. An old university friend of mine who visited during this period wittily compared the pair to a couple of old men out of a Pinter play.

Maurice informed his brother that he had to leave. One of Maurice closest friends in the latter part of his life was Sidney Corob. With his wife Elizabeth, he lived just up the road from the Vale of Health and were members, like Maurice, of the Hampstead Synagogue. Elizabeth and Sidney had started up a rather exclusive Jewish home for the elderly, and it was they who rode to the rescue to find a room for A.D. He was very happy there.

In her 2011 interview with Allan Gaw, Helen Bamber wonders about Pappworth's loneliness in old age. She astutely observed that he 'didn't belong to an old boy network'. That wasn't the Pappworth way. Bamber also showed great insight when she made the distinction that he was 'not lonely so much as cursed with aloneness,' admitting that this 'haunted' her. She continued: 'I think anybody who is against the established order of the day, who does not toe the line, who is outspoken and critical, is bound to be alone.' Bamber remembered her final image of Pappworth. She had been to visit him at Vale Lodge and, when she left, had to climb the hill that led up to the bus stop. As she mounted, she turned round and watched him go back towards the house. 'I thought then how alone this man is – this small figure limping… down the hill.'

After he died, I found among my father's papers some jottings from his solitary hours. Always an enthusiast for quotations, he had amassed a kind of literary accompaniment to the griefs over which, in his 'aloneness', it was all too easy to brood. One comes from *King Lear*, Shakespeare's searing tale of three daughters' relationship with their father: 'How sharper than a serpent's tooth it is/ To have a thankless child!' Scrawled on another scrap of paper, I found a reassurance that 'Even bad marriages can produce good children.' He threw nothing away.

'When doctors get sick': the physician as patient

The time was approaching when Maurice Pappworth needed to put his affairs in order. As a physician who had always taken a particular interest in coronary disease, he recognised the deterioration of his own condition. Since the age of sixty-three, when he first observed signs of dyspnoea (shortness of breath) climbing two hundred yards up the steep incline on Hampstead Heath just outside his house, he realised he was suffering from a heart condition. In July 1981, he experienced his first myocardial infarct: the technical term for a heart attack, when blood flow stops to a part of the heart causing damage to the heart muscle. It is generally the result of coronary artery disease. When, in 1973, Pappworth first experienced his dyspnoea, Dinah (later to become a midwife) was the only one of his children to whom he broke the news. He would have felt that her strength of character and fine brain – more scientifically inclined than her sisters' – made her better able to absorb things. It was she who noticed him stopping on the long haul up the hill as we walked home from synagogue, ostensibly to point out something of interest but in fact seizing the chance to slip a magic little pill under his tongue: glyceryl trinitrate (GTN).

Maurice's disease remained well-controlled for more than ten years. But eventually he became a regular patient at the nearby Royal Free Hospital, treated (at his request) by the distinguished cardiologist and fellow Liverpool alumnus Dr Tom Evans. I can remember some of the heart attacks and false alarms which launched him into a bed on the hospital ward. In July 1981, Maurice hosted in his fairly large garden the Vale of Health Society's celebration of the royal wedding of Prince Charles and Princess Diana. There was a barbecue; there were – heaven forbid – pork sausages. Maurice seems to have spent most of the party rushing around ensuring that no-one brought this 'treifah' food inside his house.

The outcome of his loyalty to crown and neighbours was a myocardial infarction, although this is the family's version of events. The testimony of his son-in-law Buck is invaluable; he and Dinah were staying at Vale Lodge when this first full heart attack occurred. He vividly remembers that garden party, with Maurice 'very happy in his role of host'. At about 10.30pm, he and Dinah, in the bedroom opposite, heard 'a muffled voice, or in hindsight a groan, emanating from Maurice's bedroom,' and 'it became very clear that he was in great distress'. Buck managed to find the GTN his father-in-law requested, and Dinah slipped the pill under his tongue.

When they proposed calling an ambulance to take him to the Royal Free, he refused to co-operate, but did suggest they call his friend and neighbour Dr MacPherson. 'As expected, he was a little inebriated and incoherent' – but turned out to be 'really good with Maurice'. It was 'Mac' who persuaded him to accept transport to the hospital by car and remained with him during the admissions procedure. 'Maurice was unable to walk,' recalls Buck. 'I could hear him recite the *Shema* [traditionally recited by a Jew at the point of death] over and over as I carried him downstairs'. It was once he had been admitted to the Royal Free that our father suffered the actual myocardial infarction, which he survived. This would certainly not have been the case had he been on his own at home. On the Friday night, Dinah and Buck were at his hospital bedside to light the Sabbath candles. 'It was very moving, and my father-in-law had tears in his eyes.' Maurice's own version of the story, as we shall find out shortly, was rather different.

July 1990 found me watching the penalty shoot-out between England and Germany in the World Cup semi-final. As a child, I had enjoyed watching football and tennis on television with my father. By his side in his 'study,' I watched England win the World Cup in 1966. Now, twenty-four years later, I felt my heart pounding as I watched the shoot-out and told myself that I needed to telephone my father. Predictably, he had been watching the match; predictably, his heart was also on overdrive. He was in north London; I was in Tonbridge, Kent, with two toddlers. There was little I could do except talk calmly to him and say that he should call an ambulance.

That turned out to be a false alarm. On those occasions when I was already in Hampstead, or able to get here swiftly, the main problem was trying to help the ambulance driver find the house, which was almost at the end of the road and concealed by a high garden wall. It always seemed to be dark. Like all doctors, Maurice hated being a hospital patient. 'Keep away from doctors,' he used to advise me. When he went into hospital he comforted himself with two special items. We learned to anticipate the ritual of placing these in the overnight bag which, like a woman reaching the end of her pregnancy, he kept always to hand. His own pair of down pillows and the siddur – Jewish prayer book – were all that he required.

It was a piece of advice given by my father's rabbi that, along with Anthony's conversion through a Reform synagogue, made me decide to turn my back on the Orthodox Judaism in which I had been raised. The whole incident was a re-run of the identical advice offered to Naomi twenty years earlier, which in her case sealed her rejection of her Jewish faith. In both cases the question for the rabbi was 'My father loves going to the synagogue on Shabbat, but he has a heart condition, and can no longer walk up the hill on the way home. Surely it is acceptable to be driven there and back in a car?' Both rabbis gave the same answer: 'No.' It was against the rules of the Sabbath even to be a passenger in a car. Better that he stay at home and pray on his own. My father often did this, and derived much comfort from mumbling through the service at his own pace seated in his Eames armchair.

But just as much as spiritual comfort, he needed company. Synagogue was not just a religious edifice but a meeting place (the meaning of its Hebrew name, 'Beit Haknesset'): a place to talk to friends after the service, and sometimes during it. Pappworth loved talking. To deprive him of it on the grounds of a religious law laid down long before the invention of the internal combustion engine was insensitive, even cruel – though I do remember that rabbi as generally a wise and gentle man. Once again, Sidney Corob stepped in, providing a chauffeur-driven service to the synagogue whenever required. It says much that Maurice chose to accept the kindness of a friend rather than the advice of a rabbi.

The most dramatic heart attack occurred not long before he died. Dr Pappworth had been invited to deliver a lecture to the Jewish Medical Association. In a moment still vividly remembered by those who witnessed it, the speaker collapsed, mid-sentence, on the podium. Pappworth had always insisted that he did not wish to be resuscitated in these circumstances. However, there is little hope of such a choice being respected when you collapse in front of an audience of Jewish doctors. Rushing *en masse* to the stage, they successfully set about re-starting his heart. His chief complaint to me afterwards concerned the pain that resulted from his saviours breaking several ribs in the process.

Towards the end of his life, Pappworth contributed a chapter to a book called *When Doctors Get Sick*. Edited by Harvey Mandell and Howard Spiro, it was published in 1987 by Plenum Medical, New York. The book consisted of a series of essays, all by doctors, of their own experiences of being ill. It was a clever concept: to show the doctor at the receiving end. Doctors, as is well-known, make poor patients. Pappworth, who contributed a chapter on 'Coronary Disease', was described by a reviewer on BBC Radio Four as 'the star of the book'. His account of his symptoms and treatment when his condition started to deteriorate is not hard to follow.

Pappworth was quick to spot small details: for example, the GTN which he dissolved under his tongue to relieve chest pain and as a prophylactic prior to exertion tended to lose its potency *before* the expiry date on the bottle. All proposed drug therapy he, naturally, questioned. He was not at all keen on beta-blockers, as his blood pressure had always been well within normal limits. 'I was sceptical about the suggested value of these drugs in preventing subsequent myocardial infarction, and regard the phrase "cardiac protective" as a sales gimmick.' He continues, however: 'But I had made up my mind to be an obedient and compliant patient.'

So he took the beta-blockers. These drained him of all energy. After discussion with a GP friend, he discontinued the tablets. 'Two days later, on the 29 of July 1981, although I spent the whole day sitting in my garden and later watching a long television programme on Prince Charles's wedding, I developed pain in the region of both sterno-clavicular joints radiating to the shoulders. GTN did not relieve the pain, which gradually increased in intensity.' Unless the Vale of Health party in the Pappworth garden took place the day, or the weekend, before the royal wedding, this account is very different from Dinah and Buck's first-hand version of events.

'For the first time in my life,' confesses Pappworth, 'I had great anxiety about my physical condition.' He asked his GP for advice, which was to go straight to hospital. He was eventually sent from Accident and Emergency at the Royal Free to the Coronary Care Unit. Pappworth experienced what many patients, all too quickly, discover when you face a long wait in A & E. What particularly upset him was the registrar's insistence that he go for a chest X-ray. This meant getting up from his couch and walking thirty yards to the X-ray department. As a result, Pappworth experienced severe pain which 'made me call out for help'. For the first time 'in my long medical career I appreciated precisely what physicians of a former generation had meant by the term *angor animi* – which may be translated as a patient's perception that he is dying.'

The registrar informed him that the ECG showed changes indicating a myocardial infarct. It was 3am: time for bed in the coronary care unit with pain relief via intravenous heroin. First thing the following morning, Pappworth's determination to be an obedient patient was once more put to the test when the registrar announced, 'I want to twist your arm and get you to agree to a thallium scan.' Pappworth records, 'I wanted to cry out as Job had done, "Cease and let me alone."'

When the registrar said it would be 'interesting' to see what the thallium scan showed, that remark was a red rag to a bull. 'I informed him that I have always been strongly opposed to submitting any patient to an investigation solely on the grounds that the result might be "interesting."' Tom Evans explained that this particular registrar, although he was poor at relating to patients, was nevertheless an expert at inserting pacemakers. Pappworth 'expressed my opinion that I preferred a genuine clinician to a medically qualified plumber'.

He was indeed seeing life from the other side of the screen. His experience brought home to him how frightening the 'paraphernalia' of hospital admission can be to a seriously ill patient. He recalls that the apparatus for cardiac resuscitation was kept in the corridor outside his room, 'and the noise of the sudden scurrying of the staff and the ringing of alarms and telephones disturbed the slumber I craved'. This will be familiar to many, as will the doling out of night-time drugs when the patient is already asleep, and the early-morning wake-up call for drugs and observations.

Pappworth was admitted three more times to the Royal Free between his 1981 myocardial infarction and the publication of *When Doctors Get Sick* in 1987 – although there were to be more before his death in 1994. In each account of his admission, he records how long he had to wait in A & E. On one occasion, the doctor was so nervous about having to examine the great Maurice Pappworth that he carried out a physical examination of anxiety-producing thoroughness, which included the testes. Pappworth was put on a drug which caused severe bladder retention, and encouraged to get out of bed to try and relieve his bladder while being supported by a nurse. His account of what followed is typical of the kind of detail Pappworth was not afraid to mention: 'It was usually the most attractive nurse who agreed to that procedure, but several times this had embarrassing consequences which made urination even more difficult.' So the staff resorted to catheterization, which led to him painfully passing 'red-hot razor blades' several times an hour.

Pappworth notes that his fourth admission arose from his waking in the night with 'palpitations and slight retrosternal discomfort and feeling rotten'. The word 'discomfort' was one used frequently by our father, and is typical of the stoical attitude to illness which seems to have run throughout the Pappero-vitch family. He really meant that he was suffering from outright pain – some-times very severe. Now that I am afflicted with a heart condition myself, I can understand how courageous he was in dealing with this pain and the sharp cur-tailment of a busy life – and how much he spared us. Pappworth himself main-tains, 'I am by nature an optimist and have always regarded, until recently, my own aches and pains as of no significance.'

It wasn't until I read his own account of heart disease that I realised that, in addition to feeling lethargic and weak, he suffered during the mid-1980s from anorexia. He certainly became noticeably thin, and had never had much flesh on his bones. He wondered to himself whether these symptoms were caused by the cardiac lesion or by the drugs. Once his drugs had been gradually reduced, his condition improved. This difficulty, 'perhaps impossibility', of differentiat-ing clearly between symptoms due to drugs and those due to the illness itself was, Pappworth concluded 'One of the main lessons I have learned from my illness.' Symptoms such as vertigo, headache, lethargy and gastro-intestinal problems should not be 'lightly dismissed' by doctors, as they 'make the patient miserable and despondent and might delay recovery. Drugs can easily convert the most rational and intelligent of patients into hypochondriacs.'

Pappworth's essay in *When Doctors Get Sick* concludes with two striking but very different points. He reminds his predominantly American readers of the value of the British National Health Service: his hospital admissions 'did not cost me a cent and would not have even if I were not a physician'. He em-phasises his strongly-held belief that doctors, their spouses and their children should never be charged by their colleagues for medical services. His other final topic is even closer to his heart: the Jewish philosophy which had taught him to be 'more concerned with the immediate future than any hereafter'. His adher-ence to Orthodox Judaism had, he hoped, 'inspired me to attempt to make this world, even to the slightest degree, a better place than when I arrived in it.'

Pappworth was stimulated to follow up issues that the book had brought to the fore. For example, he had written to his consultant asking if he could be given access to his patient records, which might act as an *aide-memoire*. The answer was a flat 'no'. At the time, this was forbidden. Pappworth cut out and put inside his copy of *When Doctors Get Sick* an article in the *BMJ* in September 1987. It announced that anyone would in the near future be entitled to access their personal data by making a written request and paying a fee; this included their medical records. Unfortunately, when eventually passed, the Access to Health Records Act 1990 allowed access only to medical records written on or after 1 November 1991. Once more, Pappworth had spotted an infringement of individual rights which came to be corrected.

The brutal onset of old age sent out other warning signs. After reversing in the dark into a skip (he complained it wasn't bearing the statutory warning lamp) and then driving his automatic Vauxhall estate into the garage, pressing the wrong pedal and reversing out at high speed straight into his neighbour's car, Maurice realised that a lifetime's driving had come to an end. It can be a watershed: that moment when you realise that you are no longer fit to drive, and have thus lost an important aspect of independence and control. More seriously, Esther – the sibling who had shown him the most affection and support – died in April 1992. Having used the National Health Service all her life, when she was diagnosed with heart disease in her eighties she decided to become a private patient so that she could be looked after by her brother's cardiologist, Tom Evans. Compared to Maurice's and Naomi's, her heart disease was of short duration. She was eighty-six when she died, Naomi at her bedside, a month after the birth of our son Adam. So Maurice was even more alone.

A year after Esther's death, and it was time once more for Passover. Maurice knew the time had come to go some way towards righting wrongs. He continued to refuse any contact with Jean, but he did make up his differences with Naomi, just as he and Sidney now found themselves more or less reconciled. It was fourteen years since A.D.'s death in San Francisco. With Esther's passing, Maurice had lost the one sibling to whom he felt close.

Spring 1994 found him eagerly anticipating a visit over Passover from Dinah and her three sons. They now lived in Dallas, having settled there when Buck decided that Israel was not for him. For Jewish families, the Seder night dinner is, like Christmas lunch, a time for everyone to get together. It had always been a key moment of the year during our childhood. Our father would plan out well in advance who was to read what, allowing precedence to the children – usually eight of us. So it was that at Seder night 1994 Maurice Pappworth met the three grandsons he had never seen: one because he had been born in Texas only just over a year earlier, the other two because their grandfather had chosen to have nothing to do with them or their parents. Their father Nick had not been invited. I remember it as an occasion that, despite its happy assembly, was fraught with a slightly desperate urgency. We all knew it would be our last Seder night with our father. It simply had to be a success; an entire album of photos needed to be taken. Dinah's three sons called him 'Saba', the Hebrew name for 'Grandpa', which he loved. Only his two oldest grandchildren – possibly – remember him today.

Better late than never: Fellowship at last

Pappworth had responded to his blackballing by the Royal College of Physicians with a two-fingered gesture. In an article for *World Medicine* in November 1980, he declared with his characteristic blend of confrontation and humour: 'If the medical establishment consider that they have gained revenge against me by such exclusion, and if this has made them happy, then I proclaim, "Good luck to them," because I have always favoured the spreading of happiness. Rather than moaning and indulging in self-pity because I am not a Fellow, I rejoice that I am not of that large undistinguished multitude but belong to a very select band of less than ten who have been Members without the Fellowship for over forty years.' He followed this bravado, two fingers still in the air, by toasting 'A fig to the Fellowship!' Pappworth claimed that, if offered it, he would not accept, citing the precedent set by the famous nineteenth-century pathologist Thomas Hodgkin when he refused the FRCP blazon because it had become debased.

But, as many of his admirers agreed, it was a scandal. Routine practice was for physicians to be awarded a Fellowship of the College ten to fifteen years after passing their Membership exam, but the brilliant Dr Pappworth, who had gained his MRCP in 1936 and was now in his eighties, had not been made a Fellow. This injustice was, according to Professor Martin Gore, 'very personal stuff'. Then, at surprising speed, a change in attitude started to emerge. Sir John McMichael of the Hammersmith Hospital, severely criticised in *Human Guinea Pigs*, died in March 1993. Sir Christopher Booth, another establishment figure whom Pappworth had alienated, and who had penned probably the most negative review of *Human Guinea Pigs*, seemed to mellow considerably and become something of an admirer.

Booth was a distinguished gastroenterologist and, like McMichael, a former director of the Royal Postgraduate Medical School at the Hammersmith. Described by Stephen Lock in his 2012 obituary in the *BMJ* as a man who 'never bore grudges', Booth entered into some positively amicable correspondence with Pappworth, even arranging to meet him for tea. Booth has been described as a 'difficult character to judge', with possible traces of anti-Semitism, but outwardly he appeared to have achieved a convincing *volte face*. It was he who was to write Pappworth's obituary for the *BMJ*. Booth was now the College's Harveian librarian.

One of Pappworth's chief enemies at the College, and its Registrar from 1975, was Dr David Pyke, a diabetics specialist. One interviewee assured me that Pyke 'hated' Pappworth. His personal antipathy was grounded chiefly in what he considered Pappworth's undermining of the value of the Membership by giving candidates tips beforehand about likely questions. In 1993, when Professor Leslie Turnberg became President of the Royal College, Pyke retired. A very conservative and also powerful man, Pyke would consider the list of proposals for the Fellowship and stamp them *fiat* or *non fiat*. Although Council was allowed to see the final list, what the Registrar said mainly went.

With Pyke's departure, the last obstacle to Pappworth becoming a Fellow of the Royal College of Physicians had been removed. Leslie Turnberg, now President, was a supporter of Pappworth and a fellow Jew originally from Manchester. Soon after starting in his new post, Turnberg despatched Dr Barry Hoffbrand (as the latter recalled in interview) to cross Hampstead Heath from his home in Highgate to visit Pappworth, and check in person whether he would accept the offer of a Fellowship. Pappworth was, apparently, 'very pleased'. Turnberg was delighted to be taking the lead in 'correcting what seemed to me to be an injustice so long'.

So, at the age of eighty-three in March 1993, fifty-seven years after gaining his MRCP, Pappworth received a letter from the College Registrar, David London, giving 'formal notification that Council wishes to nominate you for election to the Fellowship'. In these special circumstances, London adds, 'I very much hope that you will accept, as I know that to see your name in the lists would delight your many friends and admirers, and would serve as a public acknowledgement of your contribution to Medicine.'

The anger melted away. Pappworth said 'Yes'. Turnberg remembers clearly Pappworth's 'obvious delight' in accepting, 'without any rancour'. The Registrar wrote to Pappworth again at the end of the month, expressing great pleasure at his acceptance and noting that 'I have very happy memories of your excellent Membership classes'. He and Turnberg were unhappy about the way people were elected to the Fellowship. David London believed that people like Pappworth were 'badly mishandled... There was a gross injustice.'

The time was clearly ripe for the awarding of Pappworth's Fellowship. A letter of congratulations from Dr Gareth Beevers, a former MRCP student, mentions that he had in fact proposed some years earlier that Pappworth be made a Fellow, but that David Pyke refused to consider it. 'I was angry and upset,' admits Beevers, 'and ashamed that the ghastly College men were still as small-minded as they have been for centuries.' Another doctor described the College as a 'very constipated' institution. In the early 1990s invitations were still being written in Latin. Concluding his letter, Beevers assured his old teacher that 'you have done more for British Medicine than practically all the silly old grey tops who hang around the College, using it as an excuse not to do their out-patient clinics!' Similarly, a letter of congratulations from a doctor at Stoke Mandeville Hospital revealed that he also had written to the College on the Fellowship question, and had 'personally tackled the President head on... but got nowhere'. He continues, 'What you have done with regard to making life safer and better for the patients... will be remembered long after your detractors have passed on.'

A letter from Stephen Lock, a former student who at the time was editor of the *British Medical Journal* and later wrote Pappworth's only obituary in a national newspaper, reinforces claims for Pappworth's contribution to British medicine to be recognised by the RCP. He expresses his delight that Pappworth had been 'magnanimous enough to accept the restitution'. Michael O'Donnell, a physician who became well-known through his journalism and television appearances, described Pappworth's Fellowship as 'a sunbeam of enlightenment' that had eventually 'pierced the fog that enshrouded the RCP'.

Pappworth predictably received a snowdrift of letters expressing delight at the 'better late than never' news of his election. Many of these came, naturally, from the doctors who had benefited from his 'inspirational' postgraduate teaching. Pappworth seems to have kept all of these, and visible on some of them are the teacher's handwritten notes on their current places of work. It must have given Pappworth great pleasure to receive a letter of congratulations and gratitude from Melbourne; he had always had a soft spot for his Australian students.

At one point it looked as if Dr Pappworth might not be well enough to attend the ceremony. In this instance, the culprits were not his heart but his eyes. The problem, diagnosed as hyperthyroidism, started towards the very end of his life, and was never entirely resolved. He was assured that the condition would improve over time, but it clearly troubled him a great deal. His eyes were watering, and he was unable fully to open one of them. He didn't live long enough to experience the promised improvement. But fortunately, he was able to attend the ceremony at the Royal College on 2 June 1993. My father didn't suggest that I go as his guest. Instead, he was accompanied Dr Mary Bliss. Writing to me after his death, she explained how, incensed by the College's refusal to give Pappworth a Fellowship, she had decided to refuse it should it one day be offered to her. She had kept to her word until there was an 'unusual happy ending', when both of them were offered the Fellowship in 1993.

None other than Christopher Booth led the spontaneous applause at the ceremony as Pappworth went up to receive the award. Writing to the newly-created Fellow afterwards, Registrar David London declared, 'I have been to a number of Fellowship ceremonies and this was the only one where I have heard spontaneous applause.' He told me in interview how proud he was of his part in awarding Pappworth the Fellowship: 'I regard it as one of the best things I did in medicine,' adding 'It was very gracious of him to accept.'

When London told me about the ceremony, there were tears in his eyes. 'This little man shuffled up to get his Fellowship, and applause (led by Christopher Booth) broke out… It was very moving… A wrong was being righted.' Helen Bamber was similarly moved when she heard about this 'standing ovation… the arc of his life from being an outsider and also a very brilliant young doctor, then being separated from everything – then finally, in a way, being recognised at least in his own lifetime.' He obviously enjoyed the event. Turnberg describes him after the ceremony 'sitting at the top table at dinner in the evening. He was of course a twinkly old man by then.' His blue eyes did indeed twinkle when he was happy. Those eye problems don't seem to have been afflicting him on this occasion. It is a great pity that none of his family was there. I suspect that I was being punished for not inviting him to my D.Phil. graduation ceremony at Oxford twelve years earlier, fearful as I was of him clashing with my mother. Typically, our father had underplayed his personal story at this moment of triumph.

Farewell to 'the best teacher that ever was'

It had become part of the routine that I always telephoned my father on a Friday evening: Erev Shabbat. After the birth of our third child it became increasingly difficult to make the journey from Bromley, where we lived, but even a phone call could be a highlight for him. I had kept in touch with Herbert Samuels, son-in-law of Maurice's cousin Minnie. He and his wife Dorothy were enormously kind to me when I made my first trip to New York in 1973, and I had kept in touch with them. Herbert, now widowed, loved Britain, and used to visit from time to time. He was due to arrive, and to stay with us in Bromley, on 12 October 1994. So that week I rang my father a few days earlier than usual, on the Tuesday evening. We needed to sort out when I was going to bring Herbert up to Hampstead. My father was as talkative as ever, his main concern being Herbert's proposed trip to the Lake District. 'It's October. It will be cold up there. He's got a heart condition, remember.'

That was the last time I ever spoke to my father. Herbert duly arrived, and we entertained him for dinner along with our sister-in-law, Sue. At about half-past nine the telephone rang. Anthony took the call. It was one of my father's neighbours, who opened with the words 'I was so sorry to hear about your father-in-law.' I overheard none of this. Anthony eventually ascertained that the neighbour who found Dad had, in the first instance, telephoned Jean with the news. As they were not divorced, Jean was technically his next of kin. In any case, his sensitive neighbour may have realised that our mother would be better able than her daughters to take the blow.

After we had finished dinner, Anthony took me downstairs to the children's playroom and told me that my father had died. He says the howl I uttered was something primeval, a sound he had never heard before. But for a man who dreaded hospitals, to die in his sleep in the middle of the night was the right way to go, although I still worry sometimes that it may have been in a moment of sudden agony that he left this world. The neighbour who found him (she into whose car he had reversed) couldn't have been kinder. On the evening of 12 October, he had been due to host a meeting of the Vale of Health Society. Receiving no answer when they rang the bell, his fellow committee-members decided to let themselves in; Mrs Prasard held a key to Vale Lodge. She entered the dark hall of a house that seemed completely empty. So she ventured upstairs, and there he was.

Maurice Pappworth was buried at Bushey Cemetery, the ever-expanding resting place for the United Synagogue dead. He had made it clear that he didn't want an autopsy performed (another breach of Jewish law) but his wishes had to be disregarded, as the death was sudden. His memorial service at the Hampstead Synagogue was conducted by the Reverend Isaac Levy, its former minister: chaplain to the Jewish Forces during the war and one of the first to enter the Bergen Belsen camp. He was always a friend whom our father admired enormously. The eulogy was given by Dr Barry Hoffbrand, who features in this book.

An obituary by Stephen Lock, editor of the *BMJ*, appeared in *The Independent* on 12 November. He opens by quoting John Pearson's explanation of the eccentric Osbert Sitwell and applying it to Maurice Pappworth: 'Perhaps he was congenitally angry as some are congenitally deaf or asthmatic.' Lock goes on to record the results of this 'campaigning vehemence': today, he writes, patients are 'protected by having to give informed consent to any procedure not strictly for their benefit, while study protocols have to be approved by local research ethics committees'.

Lock recalls the way that his *BMJ* predecessors, and other medical editors, had often rejected Pappworth's letters on unethical medical research. He floats the theory that Pappworth may have been a victim of anti-Semitism, but acknowledges that a chief reason for his failure to find a consultancy job in London is that he was always a 'quintessential outsider'. The obituary observes that he 'did not mince his words' and maintained an 'acerbic view' of the Royal College of Physicians as 'a stuffy élitist club'. Lock highlights Pappworth's 'outstandingly successful' MRCP classes, which led him to be acknowledged not only as 'the best medical teacher in London, but probably throughout Britain'. He also makes the important point that Pappworth went public 'at a time when authority was being questioned and there was a revulsion against science after the thalidomide tragedy and the publication of Rachel Carson's book *Silent Spring*'. The obituary concludes with a celebration that, after fifty-seven years, 'the wounds were healed' and Pappworth was awarded his FRCP to spontaneous applause. This tribute, according to Lock, 'testified not only to the relief that good sense had prevailed on both sides, but also that honour was at last being done to a man who, however challenging and prickly, had done medicine and the wider world considerable service.'

In his December obituary in the *BMJ*, Pappworth's former foe Christopher Booth echoed Lock's reference to the 'vehement campaigning', which made

Pappworth more responsible for the increased respect for patients' interests 'than anyone of his time in Britain'. Booth also cited the notorious 'no Jew could ever be a gentleman' story, and pointed out that the job for which Pappworth had unsuccessfully applied went to the first person whom he had successfully coached for the MRCP examination. In January 1995, an obituary in the *Jewish Chronicle* stressed the influence of the Jewish ethical viewpoint on Pappworth's attitudes to human experimentation, and mentioned his conversations on ethics with Chief Rabbi Lord Jakobovits and Dr Isaac Levy, who officiated at his memorial.

Many letters of condolence were sent to me individually. They provided enormous comfort, and showed me how important it is to make a point of writing to the bereaved. There were, of course, the personal ones, some from friends of our father's, some from neighbours and fellow congregants. They remembered his wit, his provocative comments, his charm, his 'sweet and amusing' character.

There were many, naturally, from doctors. Among these was one from Dr Patricia Laird, a former MRCP student of his, who recalled Pappworth's habit of pronouncing 'exam' as 'eggzam'. Stephen Lock wrote after I had thanked him for his obituary, mentioning his pleasure that that Maurice Pappworth's papers were to be placed in the archives at the Wellcome Institute for Medical History. He also expressed his ambition that Pappworth should have an entry in the *Dictionary of National Biography*. One correspondent declared that she had the *Primer of Medicine* beside her as she wrote: 'Very few medical books are as clear as his, and none that I've found have been as much fun to read.'

There were letters also from doctors abroad. Our father's friend Dr Eli Davis, of the Hadassah Hospital in Jerusalem, wrote to commiserate after reading the obituary in the *BMJ*. He referred to Maurice by his Hebrew name of 'Moshe' (Moses), rarely heard since his childhood. Davis wrote that 'He was a fine Jew and a true family man... generous, agreeable, a wonderful host, a real doctor who emphasized the importance of learning from a patient clinically before proceeding to tests. The profession and Jewry are the poorer without him.' From New York came a letter written by our father's old friend and collaborator, Dr Dennis Bloomfield, with whom the proposed layman's guide to cardiology was to have been written. He noted that in Pappworth's death the profession 'loses just about the best teacher that ever was'.

Reading these letters, one cannot resist wondering whether, in some ways, Maurice found advantages in living without Jean. Bloomfield's letter, and those of two former Australian MRCP students, remember genuine hospitality at Vale Lodge. They also suggest that Maurice could, in his final years, be more relaxed about entertaining friends and colleagues than when he needed to take into account his wife's rather inconsistent responses to house guests.

For me, one of the most moving letters of condolence came from Joyce Allwood. Her husband, Dr William Muirhead, had before the war been a medical officer in Surrey, and met Maurice Pappworth when the latter worked at St Helier Hospital in Carshalton. Maurice used to visit the couple at their home in Banstead, but this 'happy relationship' was interrupted when both men joined the RAMC.

Demobbed in August 1946, William Muirhead returned home gravely ill. His widow's story speaks volumes about Pappworth's generous nature: 'I sought your father. We had not met for some years but Maurice came at once – not easy for him – he had no car. He was assiduous and unstinting in his care of my husband, who sadly died in St Helier Hospital in October 1946. I was pregnant with my second child – my parents lived far away – this was not Maurice's problem but he quietly took over – he handled all correspondence with [the] Ministry of Pensions – he arranged for me to be attended by one of his colleagues. My son was born in St Helier Hospital January 1947, everything organised by your father. He visited me at least once every day, entertaining me with his witty conversation – always bringing a small gift of interesting reading matter. It was a terrible time in my life made so much more bearable by your father's efforts. He was a man of great intellect, but quietly and unobtrusively he was also a man of very deep caring and compassion. I have never forgotten nor ceased to be grateful for his support.'

Mrs Allwood goes on to mention her son, William Muirhead-Allwood, whom I remember well. When he was a medical student at St Thomas's, he used to come to the Pappworth home for dinner from time to time. It was a great treat for the three daughters to entertain this tall, good-looking young man, though I fear that our infatuation led to some tactless teasing that must have made him blush. William became an orthopaedic surgeon, specialising in surgery on the hand. When my husband became Master of Wellington College, I discovered that this object of our adolescent interest was an alumnus of the school, but I never re-encountered him.

Conclusion

The Pappworth legacy: compassion, courage, attention

'There is little doubt that this whistle-blowing man was responsible for a major change in the way we go about research on patients.'

(Professor Leslie Turnberg, Lord Turnberg, former president of the Royal College of Physicians)

What were Maurice Pappworth's most significant achievements, and to what extent is his life's work still relevant today? His legacy falls chiefly into three areas: clinical diagnosis and the doctor-patient relationship, medical education and, of course, ethics, with specific emphasis on patients' rights. Pappworth was a great diagnostician because he could read the signs. For years, he practised what one doctor I spoke to described as 'proper general medicine'. He was, as another put it, 'a great one for the laying on of hands'. Now, with medicine so compartmentalised into different specialities, there is far less scope for practising as a general physician.

What Pappworth experienced professionally in the late 1920s and during the 1930s, before antibiotics entered the scene, was significant. When he first started practising medicine, diagnostic tools were limited. Despite huge leaps forward in the development of diagnostic technology, what some might call 'old-fashioned' clinical examination and diagnosis are still important, especially in those parts of the world where, for example, scans are not available. And at a small district general hospital that lacks the necessary equipment, the doctor still has to be able to work out quickly whether the patient needs to be sent on to another hospital. Neurologists will still do a proper neurological examination, even though they know the patient's head will later be put in a scanning machine. History-taking continues to be important, though there is less emphasis nowadays on 'the story'. Since MRI and CT scans became widely used during the late 1980s, some claim that traditional skills such as, for instance, how to oscillate or do percussion are becoming obsolete. It is such doctors, naturally, who end up failing to engage in conversation with their patients.

Now, in the early part of the twenty-first century, we are suffering from some level of 'de-skilling', as one university professor admitted to me. It is worth bearing in mind that people can always be trained to carry out procedures. American doctors in particular are worried that that, for example, their colon screening procedures could be taken away altogether and handed over to others, who would carry them out more cheaply.

So the everyday medical practice in which Pappworth believed has never entirely been gazumped – even during this most optimistic era for medicine's possibilities. The situation for many patients, despite all the bright new scanners and sophisticated histopathology, is that they are unlikely to have a diagnosis within forty-eight hours. This can be blamed on the delaying effects of the in-evitable series of standard tests. It is this delay that often causes most distress to patients. Pappworth was not always able to make a swift diagnosis by means of his clinical expertise, but he would certainly have disapproved of the plethora of diagnostic investigations taking place in the twenty-first century. Now pa-tients are subjected to over-diagnosing and over-treating. Prescriptions issued have risen threefold since the turn of the millennium.

As Dr James Le Fanu put it to me, there is 'an enormous drive to "mass-medicalise" people'. Before Pappworth came along and tried to put matters right, patients were not properly informed about the nature of the research trial in which they were to participate. Now they are being given insufficient infor-mation about the side-effects of the drugs they are prescribed. Concerns about this over-reliance on technological diagnosis have meant, however, that more attention is now being paid to what is taught at medical schools.

Greater attention to the medical curriculum, and how students are assessed, still has its roots in Pappworth's drive for improvement. Like Thomas Huxley, in his 1874 Rector's address to Aberdeen University, Pappworth was scathing about an educational system which produced students '"who work to pass but not to know. They do pass but still do not know"'. In British education in gen-eral, this problem has grown steadily worse since Pappworth quoted Huxley's words in 1980. His educational philosophy would be in conflict with much that happens today, in schools and universities. But his unseen influence remains. Leslie Turnberg identifies his 'invaluable' greatness as a teacher in the way he trained 'countless doctors to practise high-quality clinical medicine'.

As for medical ethics: it is not that Pappworth invented the concept, which has been in existence for as long as doctors have. What he did achieve was to put ethical issues, with particular reference to research, sharply into focus.

Ruthless in pointing the finger at named doctors who, in his opinion, had flouted good ethical practice, he has to be admired for the courage he showed in criticising a roll-call of some of the most senior and well-respected figures of the medical establishment. The emphasis he laid on the importance of informed consent was taken up by patients themselves, and acknowledged, sometimes grudgingly, by medical researchers. Questions of patient rights and welfare moved centre stage, thanks to Pappworth. *Human Guinea Pigs* lit the blue touch paper, and re-shaped the previously cavalier attitude shown by some clinical researchers to their patients. Leslie Turnberg's comment on the book is simple and incisive: 'After it, we could not do without it.'

Human Guinea Pigs was the right book at the right time. The 1960s marked the end of the age of deference, which carried with it the old belief that doctors are like gods. Although research ethics committees would probably have come into being even without the catalyst of *Human Guinea Pigs*, Pappworth's book went a long way to speeding up the process. Professor Karol Sikora describes him as 'the first whistle-blower within the system', adding 'They didn't like him because they knew he was right.' Professor Turnberg insists, 'There is little doubt that this whistle-blowing man was responsible for a major change in the way we go about research on patients.' According to another medical professor interviewed for this book, if Maurice Pappworth turned up today, he would say 'At last they've done something about what I said.'

In the view of Robert Winston, expressed in his book *Bad Ideas?*, Pappworth's key argument in *Human Guinea Pigs* was that medicine was forgetting its duty to alleviate suffering. There is no doubt that his brave criticisms were massively valuable at the Hammersmith Hospital, where Winston had worked, and elsewhere. However, Winston goes on to point out that 'even this timely corrective had its costs, for the research carried out at Hammersmith was possibly never quite as clinically innovative afterwards because the emphasis tended to turn towards laboratory-based research rather than clinical trials which might have been thought ethically questionable in some way'. Winston shares Pappworth's concerns on the way modern medicine has developed: 'Envisioning its mission as one of conquering disease with science, it has tended to foster a new breed of medical men who have often approached human suffering somewhat as if it were a problem in the laboratory. In the age of "clinical science" and the preoccupation of universities with the Research Assessment Exercise, research has tended increasingly to take precedence over cure.' These words could have streamed from the pen of Maurice Pappworth.

Although there has been much improvement on the invasive tests typical of the mid-twentieth century, the whole issue remains nuanced. Researchers still sometimes struggle to define the nature of the tests they propose. The kind of experiments that Professor Sheila Sherlock undertook at the Hammersmith, and to which Pappworth took particular exception, are no longer practised. Now the fashion is for research into genetics and neuroscience, which does not involve human subjects.

The bedside doctor may now be out of fashion, but then so is clinical science – except in the area of drug development. At Northwick Park Hospital, the Institute of Medical Research was opened in 1994, but did not prove successful in every case. It was here that, in mid-March 2006, six healthy young men became seriously unwell after taking part in a clinical trial to test a drug, TGN1412, on behalf of the American pharmaceutical company PAREXEL. It was hoped that this would prove a treatment for arthritis, multiple sclerosis and leukaemia. The subjects needed transfer to the hospital's intensive therapy unit, after they developed multi-organ failure and required round-the-clock support from the critical care team.

The worst affected lost his fingers and toes, and all the subjects of this experiment were warned that they were now vulnerable to developing cancer or auto-immune diseases as a result of their exposure to the drug. Symptoms described by the research subjects included the sensation that their brains were on fire and their eyeballs were about to pop out. Fortunately – in the short term at least – all the patients recovered, the last being discharged three months after the disastrous trial took place. The success of their lawyers in claiming damages from PAREXEL meant that the victims could afford the equipment, adaptations and assistance needed as a result of their injuries. PAREXEL eventually admitted that, as they were unsure of the precise dosage, the drug should have been trialled on one patient at a time.

The Northwick Park nightmare was in fact a research project which did follow the rules. It might well have been possible to reduce the impact of the trials, but these did conform to standard ethical procedures: it is impossible to give one hundred per cent reassurance that everything will be safe. The odd idiosyncratic reaction to a drug cannot be ruled out.

Media coverage of the Northwick Park trial led to 'Human Guinea Pigs' being chosen as the subject of *The Week* magazine's 'Briefing' page on 25 March 2006. The second paragraph of the article refers to Edward Jenner's discovery of a vaccine cure for smallpox in 1796, by deliberately infecting a young boy with cowpox and later injecting him with smallpox pus. The writer continues: 'Had Jenner done the same today, he'd have ended up in jail. But since his time the rules have got ever stricter. A key development was the publication in 1967 of Maurice Pappworth's influential *Human Guinea Pigs*, which laid down greater protection for volunteers.' The establishment of ethics committees is then touched on, as is the issue of 'informed consent'. So Pappworth's work has by no means been entirely forgotten.

What happened at Northwick Park is an important coda to Pappworth's story, for it justifies his concern that, however careful researchers learned to become, there is always the danger of some future disaster. When our Aunt Naomi heard about the scandal at the Alder Hey children's hospital in Liverpool, revealed five years after her brother's death, her response was 'Maurice Pappworth, you should be here now.' Between 1988 and 1995, more than two thousand pots were used as containers for the body parts of approximately 850 infants. Until the 1999 inquiry, the public was completely unaware that Alder Hey – and indeed other NHS hospitals, most notoriously the Bristol Royal Infirmary – were retaining patients' organs without the consent of their families. Like the parents in *Human Guinea Pigs*, who were not fully informed of the experiments on their infants, parents of the children at Alder Hey were kept firmly in the dark.

One of Pappworth's bugbears was the trend to climb the medical career ladder by publishing research, however unsubstantiated its conclusion. He would have been enraged by the antics of Dr Andrew Wakefield. In 1998, Wakefield published in *The Lancet* a fraudulent research paper lending support to the later discredited claim that colitis and autism are linked to the combined measles, mumps and rubella (MMR) vaccine. As a result of all the publicity surrounding this claim, many mothers decided against submitting their baby to the triple vaccine. Inevitably, there followed a significantly increased incidence of measles and mumps, many of which proved fatal, or caused severe and serious injuries. After an official investigation into Wakefield's 'utterly false' claims, he was in May 2010 struck off the Medical Register. His self-serving lies were described in a 2011 article as 'perhaps the most damaging medical hoax of the last hundred years'. The last straw, for Pappworth, would have been that, in order to justify his theory, Wakefield subjected autistic children to unnecessary and unpleasant procedures.

These three cases, all of which occurred after Pappworth's death, offer the important truth that, as he warned, the medical profession, journalists and the general public must continue to be vigilant. The more medical science advances, the more we need to concern ourselves with the clinical, ethical and communication issues involved. Unsavoury truths about the past are still coming to light. In August 2016, when government archives from thirty years earlier were opened, it was discovered that vulnerable children in a remand home were being used as part of a top-secret clinical trial in 1966. This was of course not reported in the medical journals, and remained an abuse that even Pappworth failed to uncover. Now, almost two decades into the twenty-first century, what Maurice Pappworth said sounds like common sense – but it must be remembered that, in his day, he was considered very radical. And it is possible that being part of 'the awkward squad' made it much easier for Pappworth to express his views. One letter congratulating him on his Fellowship described him as 'a most constant irritant'. From the irritant inside an oyster, a raw pearl is produced. Arguably, he might have made more impact if he had joined 'the club' and changed things from within. However his methods are perceived, Pappworth was indeed influential. As an eminent doctor insisted to me, 'He changed things.'

May 2017 marked the fiftieth anniversary of the publication of *Human Guinea Pigs*. It has been out of print for a long time. But Maurice Pappworth left a legacy that will continue, even when his name is forgotten. There are still many in the profession who wish to keep the flame burning. As Pappworth himself touchingly admitted to his *GP* magazine interviewer in 1977, 'For many years I felt that I had very few supporters. But today I feel I have many sympathisers. Many young doctors feel as I do on certain subjects.' The medical writer Dr James Le Fanu has since Pappworth's death worked to draw attention to his legacy: in his authoritative book *The Rise and Fall of Modern Medicine* and in articles on the art of clinical diagnosis. Writing in his *Sunday Times* column on 14 January 1997, in a piece entitled 'The Old Ways Knock Spots Off the Scanner', Le Fanu refers to 'the late Dr Pappworth' as 'one of Britain's great medical diagnosticians'. Professor Allan Gaw, of the National Institute for Health Research's Clinical Research Network, shares Pappworth's particular interest in the conduct of clinical trials, medical education and coronary heart disease, has for several years been researching the work of a man whom he greatly admires.

Pappworth was one of the last true general physicians, considered by some as the greatest doctor they ever met. Described once as the Stradivarius of the medical profession, he was, as Helen Bamber put it, 'different' from other doctors, especially in his thinking. He continues to exert an 'unseen influence' on the work of many people. Maurice Pappworth was also a whistle-blower. One doctor interested in research misconduct, who has spoken to many whistle-blowers, stressed to me that the whistle-blower is the one who suffers, and is often very damaged as a consequence of revealing the truth. Efforts are now being made to rectify this danger. In February 2016 the report of a committee chaired by Sir Robert Francis QC, responding to a request from the Secretary of State, examined the National Health Service's treatment of whistle-blowers. *Freedom to Speak Up* reads in part like the words of the late Dr Pappworth: the culture of the NHS should be one in which 'patients are always put first and their safety and quality of treatment are the priority'.

This book has emphasised Maurice Pappworth's status as an outsider. He retained this throughout his life. As an outsider, he could more readily raise the whistle to his lips. But this didn't make the anxieties and ostracism any easier to bear, once the whistle's shrill voice had filled the air.

Afterword

Our father, Maurice Pappworth.

This memoir, *The Whistle-Blower*, marks 50 years since the publication of Maurice Pappworth's highly controversial book, *Human Guinea Pigs*. That book was a detailed investigation and a harrowing record of experimental research, frequently without fully informed consent, on often very vulnerable people. In daring to blow the whistle on his colleagues, Pappworth showed great bravery, moral rectitude and not a little bloody mindedness. *Human Guinea Pigs* influenced improvements in ethical standards in medical research, and greater safeguards for human subjects. This book explores the man behind the whistleblower, written from his eldest daughter, Joanna's, perspective. It highlights other significant contributions that he made to the dissemination of good practice in medicine both through his medical textbook, *A Primer of Medicine* and for the thousands of pupils he taught and continues to influence to this day.

Parents stamp our hearts forever. Maurice Pappworth was a forceful father and he left a deep and enduring imprint. It was certainly that way for Joanna. It was no less so for us, Dinah, his middle daughter, and Sara, his youngest. So, we are delighted that our older sister, Joanna, devoted so much of the remaining energy of her last year, to writing this memoir. It was a labour of love, poignant in her need to write it and in her view of who he was.

Joanna had unwavering loyalty to him. She records in this memoir that he was a very difficult man, whose short stature, outsider status and chip on his shoulder, were challenging for those around him and for himself. Joanna did not experience his scorn or anger very much. Despite some modest young adult rebellion, Joanna was his most consistent soft spot. Our relationships with our father were distinctly rockier.

Joanna did not write a great deal about our parents' marriage, stating at one point that they were both very keen to have children. And our mother, Jean, had certainly said that herself. After all, when they got married, he was 43 and she was 30. But there was more attraction and tangled emotion than that between them. Both Maurice and Jean had struggled with parents who did not provide much loving affection. They brought their huge and separate needs with them into the marriage. Perhaps they found in each other things that they needed. However, Jean did not seem to understand Maurice and Maurice seemed to need to be cruel to Jean. They each had their own vein of strong feelings which could overflow. For his daughters, it was sometimes painful to witness.

Despite his personal challenges, Maurice Pappworth was prescient in his understanding of the pitfalls of modern medicine. The needs he highlighted for respect and empathy and for providing care for patients as individuals, are at the forefront of current discourse in healthcare. So, also, is the over-reliance on testing and technology. These were some of his issues he questioned.

All three of us daughters have lived and worked in his shadow.

I, Sara, am inspired daily by both my parents in my work as a Gallery Education Curator. This job combines my mother's passion for art with my father's passion for teaching. Like my father I enjoy the process of finding the most effective ways to communicate my knowledge and enthusiasm with those I teach. I am also often guided by his emphasis on the importance of individual ethical responsibility.

I, Dinah, am a midwife. Midwifery is a rebellious profession. It is a profession which is feminist and questioning of the medical establishment. My father is with me every day in my work. He is there on the moral high ground as I advocate for the women in my care. He is present as I listen to their stories. He is by my side as I support them in the least interventive and most respectful way that I can. I am daily thankful for his legacy.

Joanna was an incredibly engaging teacher, committing much time and tremendous skill into developing the passions of the students whom she taught. At her memorial, many were present to attest to the influence that she had on their lives. That dedication and skill was our father's legacy to her.

Index

Maurice Pappworth's family changed their surname from Papperovitch to Pappworth in 1932/33. With the exception of Maurice Pappworth himself, family members, whose life is discussed prior to this date, are under the surname Papperovitch. Family members born at a later date or who married into the family after this date are filed under Pappworth. Maurice Pappworth is filed under the surname Pappworth.